Covid-19 and the
Transformation of American Society

Jose Martinez, Ph.D.

Covid-19 and the
Transformation of American Society

Jose Martinez, Ph.D.

Academica Press
Washington~London

Library of Congress Cataloging-in-Publication Data

Names: Martinez, Jose, author.
Title: Covid-19 and the transformation of american society / Jose
Martinez
Description: Washington : Academica Press, 2020. | Includes references.
Identifiers: LCCN 2020948766 | ISBN 9781680539356 (paperback)

Dedicated to

Elizabeth, Cristina, and Sara

Contents

Introduction

First things first. Coronavirus is the contagious virus that can lead to COVID-19. COVID-19 is the acronym for the Corona Virus Disease, named in 2019, which can be fatal. The virus is a medical/physiological phenomenon. Yet herein will be discussed the various social factors exacerbating the virus and how the virus itself is causing societal change. The virus is the impetus for substantial social change for the foreseeable future. The societal factors directly and indirectly related to it such as poverty, race, class and other factors will be extensively discussed. The ramifications of the pandemic are extensive. Some might muse about whether the societal and what follows herein is related to the coronavirus. Yes, it is.

In a word, the social change stemming from the ramifications of the coronavirus is significant. It needs to be understood as comprehensively as possible. This is a concise presentation of what is germane to social change from the coronavirus. The virus is not simply a physiologically isolated medical entity. It cannot be separated from a number of societal aspects, try as some may to simply focus on the disease as exclusively relegated to the physiological.

Some brief definitions are in order: Race is not a physiological reality but a set of characteristics at various points in history that society imagines/creates and foists on some groups for particular purposes. Class is one's socioeconomic position in society, though definitions of class have also shifted. Gender is more what a given society has determined to be a set of behaviors and thinking contrived since birth (girls can be as aggressive and boys as emotional as anybody else at younger ages before society channels them in particular directions). Sociology is the large-scale study of society, which will be utilized some.

What follows is not exhaustive. It is essentially, again, a concise (not trite nor ephemeral, though) yet meaningful exploratory introduction to social change brought about by the pandemic. It presages how American society and the world is changing currently as well as thereafter. In practically all facets of life, the U.S. will never be the same. The "good ole days" are gone. In fact, there never really were "good ole days" except for some perhaps enjoyed at the expense of others.

In some ways what is occurring is revelatory of what social reality has been. In some ways the structural changes that are occurring are constructive, such as a reconsideration of consumerism, what with jobs much more precarious now and in the future. Since blacks are being affected more negatively due to the socioeconomic situation they were placed in American society, much more of society as a whole now understands them a little more, and others in society now understand each other better as well.

Not constructive as a social change is the further entrenchment of inequality. Nonetheless, as will be seen here, there are renewed efforts to address the inequality. History is being rewritten and upended as we speak. It should go without saying that there is extensive inequality in health care as well as in other aspects of society. The inequality in health care is not an isolated phenomenon. It is part and parcel of what is the case in the rest of society. That will be clearly delineated here, since many shirk from seeing this.

So much so is this the new normal, so to speak, that the older normal that was around for so long in American society is going by the wayside. Simply, most did not even know there was a name for what has been the case (the older normal), namely the theory of postmodernism in particular, as well as similar theories. Too many readers eschew theory. Theory guides us in a particular direction. It is an organizing mechanism for further exploration.

Postmodernism refers to "post," what follows after modernism. Modernism refers to the idea of the linear, of things being a particular way that those in power have portrayed. For about the last forty years postmodernism was postulated as being the other way around, formally by theorists but much more informally by most anyone else, that we look at the fragments instead, the individual parts of society and think of it all as language games without much of a reference to reality, that you make of life what you will and are responsible for it, and have "ownership" of it. In a word, everything was just a personal narrative of experience, one's as good as that of the next person.

Postmodernism ultimately and unfortunately was not just a theory in social sciences but in other areas also, such as literature and architecture. That theory and particularly an offshoot of it, cultural studies, unsuccessfully tried to focus on the subjective experience as only one's individual experience, not that of others in general, as still emphasized in the Dr. Phil shows and Oprah before that, thus obviating the more meaningful macro or large scale patterns of the experiences of many.

Coherence was anathema to pomo, as it was called for short. The actual purpose of pomo thought was to eliminate structural thinking itself in the social sense and eradicate social responsibility, etc., the latter requiring that we looking out for each other, for taxes to support that responsibility as an example, as is the case throughout much of Europe and elsewhere, or even at some points in the history of the U.S.

Well, the coronavirus did what no one person could, and without intent since a virus is not an entity with a conscience, and all in short order. For one thing, among others elaborated further herein, the virus made society think in terms of others (whether they were excited about doing so or not) because of the possibility of infection by others as well. Other related aspects of the virus came swiftly into play. They are also elaborated here. Some, such as blacks, now saw that the socioeconomic circumstances that impinged on their health were factors in their now greater vulnerability from what society had done to them historically, and hence higher rates of infections/deaths for them.

Then blacks realized that they were perhaps not only dying at a higher rate because of that but also, glaringly, because of the long history of aggression against them and killings by police. Martin Luther King was clear about the violence against them and what the overall situation was in the U.S. when he indicated that the U.S. was the main purveyor of violence throughout the world. Blacks already understood that, but the coronavirus contributed to some stark realizations. These are sociohistorical situations. They further realized that, when mitigation efforts were instigated in society to lessen the spread of the coronavirus, their unemployment rate was even higher due to their being thrown out of work and/or it being even more difficult for them to find work when businesses closed and thereafter when businesses opened.

Latinos also have high rates of infection due to the fact that they had to continue working in some jobs that were classified as essential, such in meat and poultry packing, etc., and for income survival purposes continued to work. Some of these Latinos were undocumented workers and therefore did not have much of any rights, were vulnerable, and in a word could not quite refuse to work, alongside their desperate need for income. The income of many in Mexico is dependent on the earnings of these, who remit a sizable amount of their earnings to their family in that country and elsewhere.

Therefore, these segments of society, or to be more precise soon after all of society, now saw the reality. Specifically, much of what is occurring is not due to individual factors but to social factors. As mentioned above, this has been the reality in American society throughout its history. Political leaders have always tried to downplay this, hence the popularity and dominance of postmodern theory and thinking (even by those who had never heard of postmodernism). Pomo never could address class factors, and only stated that other ways of thinking than pomo were just metanarratives, without pomo being able to critique itself as a metanarrative of its own.

Hence, postmodernism had already been declared not long ago as having faded in formal theoretical circles, though society did not get that memo and pomo was still very much alive still in society as a whole, in practice. Now it cannot sustain itself as a theoretical standpoint, formally or informally.

Many related issues are now being perceived as structural in society, as patterned. Not many will tolerate anymore the trivialization of the virus as an individualistic matter. By the same token, not many will accept as well that police brutality is a problem of some individual bad apples instead of an ethos in policing. Political leaders are thus not happy about these revelations. That is why they are horrified about what has happened as well to the economy in the U.S., which has always been that of societal factors at work anyway rather than individual, ownership ones.

Confirmation of the touted individualism, which is not the actual history of the U.S., was found in the reactions to the pandemic. In a rather proud sort of way of theirs much of the media has fallen again, as they usually do, to the mantra of "personal responsibility" which is code for blaming the victim and therefore not acting on the responsibilities all have for looking out for fellow humans.

In Texas it was emphasized that rural Texans and people in cities such as Lubbock refused to wear masks, etc., to indicate that this was a free country and that Dr. Fauci, the main immunologist in the country, should not be listened to, as Lt. Governor Patrick said he was not going to listen to him. Not only that, the organizers of the in-person Republican convention in the state, blithely said that convention attendees were to just sign a paper that it was the attendee's "personal responsibility" for what may befall him or her in the convention in regard to the coronavirus.

In a spritely reporting of all this, the media did not disclose that those "conservative, Republican, red" areas of Texas flouting the orders of the governor (whose hand was forced because of the spikes in infections) to wear masks, etc., are significantly white and older and thus declining in population. In fact, the media referred pejoratively to "liberal" cities in Texas without disclosing that the large cities are comprised more so of people of color and younger, who are increasing in population. The latter reality is also the case in a city such as New York City, and not that New York City is simply "liberal" and wrong and bad and therefore had higher rates of infection because of that, as many initially implied and some still do.

The coronavirus has re-opened the wounds in the U.S. currently which historically have never been healed nor resolved. These wounds have met their reckoning lately. Namely, there is and has always been polarization in society, and society is not a conglomeration of picturesque middle-class moderates. When push comes to shove it is now clear that those who want to maintain what they have, which has too often throughout history been that of ill-gotten goods, will even kill to do so and to maintain their ethos in society. Many police have been recorded in savagely attacking and even killing blacks, Latinos, and poor whites for no reason other than to uphold their impunity over the powerless. Now recorded also is the killing even of Black Lives Matter participants and others by whites, by gunshot, car, etc.

Since much of the mainstream media is corporate, they too have struggled recently to maintain their cherished storylines, for example, of outside agitators leading the protests and even the riots, when good reportage made it clear that it simply was a matter of local people with grievances acting/protesting in their own communities and therefore collectively throughout the country in numerous cities. Nevertheless, the protestors have gotten one step ahead of all these situations lately, putting the opposition on the defensive and the latter showing their true colors, cobbled together through violence, the true colors of much of society after all which were hidden from sight for centuries, but known to and experienced by the powerless all along.

In other words, the coronavirus is not a person or persons with intent on what it does, nonetheless the social changes from the coronavirus have occurred and have changed history irrevocably. It is not a "personal" responsibility matter, it is not the province of a person. However, decisions made by those in political office, for example, are having grave societal consequences. For that reason, the pandemic is social, by definition, in innumerable ways. Many in political office and others are duly anxious about particularly the socioeconomic changes due to the virus. Better put, they are in a panic because those changes are not only real but apocalyptic as well, and the changes are undoubtedly occurring without a probability of being rolled back in time.

In regard to a devolution to the "personal," lately President Bush II and even Oprah had insisted, in league with the upper class control of society, on what has been called the ownership society, that you own up to things, that what happens is your own doing. The purpose in putting it this way is that no one therefore will need to have anything to do with you. They say that, but then they are silent about how others made it possible for them to get where they are. Trump is a good example of someone who claims that he is a self-made real estate tycoon, when in fact he inherited many millions of dollars from his father.

President Obama did point out, though, that the highways that others built made it possible for a person to travel, the schools built by others for a person to get educated, and so forth, for one's success. No one is born fending on his or her own in the cradle and not many die later on by themselves on a death bed, nor does anyone do much in between those points alone. We only are led to believe that we create our own selves.

The coronavirus thus is interwoven throughout several aspects of society and is not simply an isolated medical entity. The media emphasizes primarily the medical as if it is disjointed from societal circumstances. What will not be found herein is a medical treatise on the virus. There is more than enough literature on the technical aspects of the virus. Much of the news either has a focus on the medical factors revolving around the coronavirus and/or on topics related to the medical, such as the epidemiology of the virus, the hotspots, etc. A number of other things instead that are societal are discussed here in relation to the coronavirus. Obviously, there will be some references to the medical aspects to a certain extent here and there.

In a word, the changes in society due to the coronavirus are cataclysmic. All facets of society are affected. Very significantly, it will be more easily perceived now how so many circumstances are related to each other, which is what follows here. There are books on inequality in health care. However, here it will be seen how the coronavirus ultimately exposed furthermore the entrenched inequality overall in society. That is much more meaningful than the more narrow approaches, important as some are.

Whether in regard to relationships, to the work situation, to socioeconomic factors, to education and a host of other things, society is different and will never be the same, regardless of those in political office and others claiming otherwise every day. They fear the transformation of society, which is most definitely occurring. Actually, it is practically the entire world that is changing alongside U.S. society. There is nothing else that has made the world almost stop still, in shock.

Both world wars, the Great Depression, 9/11, etc. did not change American society and the world as extensively as COVID-19 has and will continue to do. The virus's transformations obtained in a relatively very brief period of time and within a few months initiated the cataclysm. No one was expecting this, though obviously many in science do expect that a number of things are possible, including pandemics and what they might incur.

This pandemic is different than others, and not simply in the huge numbers of people infected and dying. It is different in its long-term social ramifications for practically everyone everywhere in the U.S. and in the world. The threat of infection permeates society, even after vaccinations which are generally not completely successful. The infection can be deadly in a short period of time, even if treatments would be available, what with the entrenched inequality in American society of who gets what treatment and when.

Essentially, therefore, the coronavirus and its consequences changed society abruptly and pervasively. Only nuclear war would be worse, and that nightmare cannot be ruled out entirely given the gratuitous saber rattling in recent history. The future is a coronavirus future that even a vaccine, treatment and testing probably will not eliminate. Estimates already indicate that many more millions of people would have been infected and a large number of them would have died without mitigation efforts. Mitigation is not completely successful and cannot be.

The very word mitigation only means lessening the impact of something. It does not mean eradicating it, though the implication by some is that only if we did have more mitigation then we would conquer the coronavirus. In the summer of 2020 it seemed to be that even with mitigation there were many times the number of people infected than what was thought to be the case. Many aspects of the virus are thus unknown and unpredictable.

Many in political office and others claim that the coronavirus has not affected their lives (as the president of Brazil boasted before he got infected), but the impact is already there. In the case of the U.S. there is much suffering due to the initial nonchalant trivialization of the disease by Trump in order not to spook the stock market, which still happened. Americans, as a result of such initial inaction, paid in blood and treasure and hereafter will, due to his effort to shield his profit system. In that he failed anyway.

Some historians recently tried to diminish this pandemic by making some sort of comparison with other calamities. They claimed that other calamities did not shatter the economic system. However, they were wrong. Those other calamities were discrete and not every person was affected by them, and certainly not immediately. It is certainly the case that not even the world wars affected every person in the U.S. immediately, and in the world not everyone was affected in the economic sense. This pandemic makes quite a number of things unpredictable throughout the world, however.

Trying to mitigate the spread of the coronavirus, noble and necessary as the effort is, in the space of just two or three months instigated a relatively swift and permanent convulsion in the U.S. and the world. So many thousands of families in this society have been devastated by the death of a loved one due to the virus, such death occurring so unexpectedly, a complete shock, from something they had not even heard about only weeks before. Many have referred to the economy being upended, but the very lives of these families and all of those around the deceased have been completely upended as well.

Parenthetically, though, Americans are not much interested in knowing about others in the world. That is what others say of the U.S., which is evident in the ignorance of American students about the world in contrast to what students in other countries know about us and the rest of the world. Many Americans imagine themselves to be isolationist or want to be isolationist. The coronavirus will definitely correct such idealism. Unfortunately, many in our society sit up and take notice about problems only when something affects them directly.

These social changes will not come about in a linear way. They will abate and intensify and thereby fluctuate, but things will not be the same. This is not just in reference to the medical aspects of infection, but much more so in regard to many other life shattering factors such as the rate of unemployment that in the space of just weeks zoomed to Depression-era levels. The very types of economic activity such as careers, jobs, services, etc., are being transformed dramatically. Relationship patterns in particular are shifting before our very eyes. Due to the fear of possible death from infection, various aspects about interactions will change and shift again even more when a vaccine, treatment and testing become commonplace. The latter things will not solve the problems associated with the coronavirus neither here nor in the rest of the world. Because localities are interrelated with other localities, states with other states and regions, and the U.S. with the other countries in the world, whatever changes occur, good or bad, will thus be uneven and increase or decrease (fluctuate).

When even one or two day care workers or children get infected or when there is an infection among the larger numbers of children in a school, for example, that will obviate a lot of progress. Quarantining may work but obviously it will throw a monkey wrench into day care, schooling, and workplaces.

It is likely that those who were in contact with an infected person will be traced and watched closely and/or quarantined as well. Not much tracing, however, has been occurring in the U.S. Some countries require quarantines for persons who travel out of state and particularly to or from some countries for fourteen days or more, regardless of whether they are infected. If they are not infected that will still cost the persons in some ways.

Some will face problems at work and elsewhere from the mere fact of having a fever, which was not a major factor before in everyday interactions and transactions. At least they will become suspects in the eyes of others. Those who coughed before will now bring public condemnation upon themselves, particularly in the cabin of an airplane where passengers cannot walk away from said person. The person who coughs may not be infected with the virus as the great majority of these persons will not be, but that is beside the point now. A sneeze may send people scurrying away from him or her in places other than an airplane (there is nowhere to run inside a plane). It does not matter anymore if it was just allergies, the person will be looked at in askance and perhaps become the target of profanities or worse if he or she did not cover the sneeze.

How all this plays out in places such as dark movie theaters is unfathomable. Said movie theaters with the audience seating shoulder to shoulder may become a thing of the past. A sneeze may instigate a stampede in a movie theater with people stumbling and tripping over each other, with movie goers demanding their money back. Streaming of movies as a substitute for going to movies may not be as profitable, with all this impacting Hollywood's bottom line.

It is almost inconceivable that the level of hooping and hollering by twenty-something year old males (and others) in the audiences of violent movies will decrease, what with (contagious?) droplets spreading exponentially to others as happens when people talk louder. The question may evolve into how many more violent movies will be produced, since these types of movies bring in much revenue, when these factors regarding the coronavirus are considered. The less violence, however, the more of a relief for a society now hunkered down at home with hopefully other genres of streaming movies.

Still, the fanatic hooping and hollering at football games will not subside. With fewer fans going to the games in the stadiums, though, the spewing of said droplets will now spread within the living room to family and friends watching the games, which is a more dangerous situation given the enclosed area.

These and other social changes are occurring now and/or will quite soon, whereas American society and the world were going about essentially business as usual, not prepared and not expecting the upending. The historical residue will manifest itself in myriad and many yet unforeseen ways. This book describes and explains many of the concurrent societal changes convulsing primarily the U.S. and provides a cohesive overview of them from what is referred to in sociology as the macro (large-scale) perspective.

Contamination of doorknobs and the various detailed medical aspects of testing are not the major focus, but the more meaningful and large-scale social aspects of the pandemic are. Very importantly the historical context of some of the more meaningful situations in society will be presented, relating that to the virus and therefore why we as a society experience what we do, and have done, throughout our history.

The pandemic signifies that there apparently is a likelihood that people in our society will be less inclined to interact with each other, or at least not engage in discussions with others in relatively physically close encounters, meetings, and so forth. Yet, it is almost a contradiction in terms when there is likely more understanding and enlightenment that is increasing as a result of protests against police brutality and related racial and class issues that had not been discussed much before. Discussions cannot all be successfully done online or in virtual settings. So we have before us a possibility of greater rapport now given the emergent racial and social issues, for example, at the same time that there develops a possibility of less rapport in everyday social interaction, what with social distancing and masks, so to speak.

Even when sociology looks at the micro (small scale) perspective it is looking at groups of people at a smaller level of analysis, comparatively. Overall things are more meaningful for people when they see what is in general going on. John's or Jane's situation, though perhaps quite interesting in its own right, is usually not representative of much of anything, though it is an outside possibility that it may be if the right (representative) person is found by sheer coincidence. That is not practical but is what the media does on the cheap instead of costlier investigative reporting of larger issues in society. That type of reporting has been cut by most media outlets.

Most definitely certain categories of people in society are affected more negatively when and if they get the virus than others and in different ways. Social patterns will be analyzed instead of the experience of one or two persons, as the media is wont to do, which they call the human interest angle, meant to grab attention and thereby sell their newspapers (newspapers were not all that financially viable before the virus) or TV and internet news to subsequently attract advertisers. The patterns for larger numbers of people and certain categories of them are much more meaningful than the unrepresentative example of one individual. This applies to pandemics also.

Most people experience suffering due to the pandemic, including the many thousands who die and eventually will do so from the virus. However, some do not experience much misery, such as those in the stock market who invest in the now ubiquitous masks, sanitizers, ventilators, gloves, acrylic cashier shields, online higher education and so forth. Some in the stock market invested heavily and the market went up once it was thought that businesses were opening up successfully, then right after fell precipitously when they realized that the virus seemed to be lingering longer than expected. Many people are asymptomatic but it has now been realized also that a number of people are in fact pre-symptomatic (not yet showing symptoms but later doing so). During that period in time they can be contagious.

Whatever the case may be at a point in time, the wealthy do not have the same problems as others, even in mundane things such as getting their toilet paper. They buy it by sending their maids to the grocery store, and at one point had their subordinates wait in long lines outside stores before opening time of grocery stores. Getting toilet paper became a monumental task to many other people. So, not only can the wealthy afford health care, they are in better circumstances in regard to many other things about the coronavirus than are the rest of the populace.

The same point about social patterns can be discerned in other matters as well, such that some categories of people and their socioeconomic circumstance make it more likely they will contract diabetes. Some categories live longer than others, seen in comparisons of males and females, and the countries which have different overall patterns regarding longevity. One of the more significant categories of differences is that of class differences, thus class warfare is said to be intensifying between the better-off and those not well off. As billionaire Warren Buffett aptly put it, his class is winning and in fact, he added, it is a rout. At another point he further elaborated on that when he said his secretary pays a higher percent of her income in taxes than he does. He should know of whence he speaks.

Racism is obviously another major factor in any deliberations about the coronavirus. The definition of racism is changing, after protests about racism in police departments and society in general. Dictionaries will now include what many sociologists categorized as racism: that one group in society, whites, have basically benefitted historically and still do in a socioeconomic sense in comparison to blacks. If blacks or Latinos would in some hundreds of years in some way in general benefit more than whites in using skin color as a proxy, then it would be possible but improbable that the situation would reverse. If a black may not like a white, that is misunderstood because that would be simply prejudice. If he or she does something against a white, that would be discrimination. The overall patterns are the significant aspect, not what one person does.

Briefly, there is a similar situation regarding gender. Overall men are thus sexist against women, and benefit from that. In classism, the wealthy benefit from their class position against the lower class. When and if the goods of the wealthy are ill-gotten they certainly do not give them up and give them to the lower class. Generally, those benefitting keep their benefits, however ill-gotten they were and too often they were and are ill-gotten. They throw Christian precepts by the wayside of loving thy neighbor as thyself, something to mumble about on Sundays.

Racism is not inherently a matter of personal intention. It is not about whether a person ever enslaved anyone. Thus, it is not a matter of the past being past us, as President George W. Bush (married to a librarian but himself word challenged) once said.

Equality, by the way, does not come about through merit. Bush was a C student and became governor of Texas, while Perry was a D student (only had two A's at Texas A&M) and likewise became governor of Texas. Trump is not a physician but as President gave medical advice to the nation. That we elect people to the highest offices who are prone to ignorance and proud of it is incredible, but it is what people in the U.S. have done. The society that voted them into office is ultimately responsible and apparently much of society is satisfied with it.

Trump's advice can lead to people dying in reference to the coronavirus, so yes this is all extremely significant. We should not abide by what he says but we do, and we as a society did so as well with Bush and Perry. It is a twisted type of leadership, all the while that society needs constructive leaders. We cannot afford anything less, particularly since we have educational systems to produce a semblance of education. In sum, those in power waylay the medical experts on the virus, and other experts in other areas as well.

In terms of equality it will be about 100 years before women will have equality in general at the rate things are going, though not in every facet of society, and we will see (whoever is still around) if women become sexist to men when and if they benefit more from their gender at that point in time and beyond. Likewise with blacks and racism, but that is a matter of hundreds of years from now when there might be equality. Looking at hundreds of years from now or even 100 years is speculation about what people will or will not do.

Likewise, what follows is not speculation but the likelihood of significant changes in society from the current coronavirus. Professional expertise in analyzing society helps instead of what Trump and others like him spout. Moreover, he is not a sociologist, but what follows is much more sociological than anything he trumpets. What follows is a window into the near future with perhaps some meaning also for the distant future. It is informative to examine what is transpiring, in order for us to understand social changes.

Chapter 1

The Service Sector

One of the sociological reasons (other than the fact that this nation's population is one of the largest in the world) that cases of infection are high is because this economy is predominantly a service sector type of employment wherein people frequently interact with others because of their occupations, in comparison to other societies. Other societies/countries are more likely to be industrial as we were in recent history or even agricultural as we were many years ago as well. In the latter type of societies people do not interact with each other all that extensively. Therefore, a contagious disease such as the coronavirus will be more devastating in a largely service type of society.

Thus, in the sociological sense most employment is service oriented, providing services to others in some way. The service sector is generally low income, with significant exceptions such as physicians and some managers who are paid more than the great majority of the others in the service sector. Even then, blacks as an example face racism in the health care field not only when they are physicians and nurses themselves, but also as patients, in addition to elsewhere in the service sector of the economy other than in health care.

A good number of those being infected are physicians, nurses, and others who may make good money, which means they have better education, health care, etc., than others but still interact extensively with various people and thereby get infected as well. Wouldn't you know it, though, that a disproportionate number of blacks and Latinos who work in health care do so in the poorer hospitals with more blacks and Latinos as patients. The same applies to black and Latino teachers who work in poorer schools. In fact, service workers are increasingly people of color, with the percentage much higher in certain occupations than in others.

There are consequences to those of color willing to work under such conditions in contrast to better-off employments. Due to racism and discrimination by employers, some people unwillingly are rather placed in those positions, to put it nicely. Then these health care workers and teachers are expected to work miracles with insufficient resources. This has already been noted by health care workers who are battling COVID-19 without adequate masks, ventilators, etc., provided for them in their settings, in contrast to the better hospitals.

Both patients and students in poor neighborhoods are already under difficult economic and other circumstances, again in contrast to those in the better-off neighborhoods. Yet the miracles are still expected from them out of nowhere. If not, those working there won't be promoted, while those working in better-off circumstances find it easier to do their job and to thus be promoted for their "good work."

The socialization of many people by society is such that even many patients and students both have become skeptical of professionals of color. The latter are questioned more, etc. The racism is palpable in just about every facet of work that those of color do. As a personal aside, that is exactly what I and most any colleague of color have found, no matter the academic background and the accomplishments a person of color has (in my case with previous books having hundreds of references), the experience, etc.

Professionals of color have to prove themselves every minute in contrast to whites who do not have to or are not even professionals, such as Trump with his outright falsehoods on the pandemic or on practically anything else, with such statements of his accepted at face value by his base, which is millions of people. There are entire books now on the experiences of professionals of color. The title of one of them about professors of color says it all: Presumed Incompetent, by Gutierrez y Muhs, Niemann, Gonzalez, and Harris.

Inequality is woven throughout all aspects of the pandemic. The reason is simply because inequality is interwoven throughout society.

There are also many who work in social agencies who thereby interact extensively with a variety of people every day. Many of these working in such agencies are people of color and do not in general get paid much. A good number of them majored in the social sciences out of a desire to help others like themselves.

Then there are those who work as police in providing services without very high pay but who are more likely in their line of work than others to interact with a diverse set of people, touching and even forcibly holding suspects and sometimes getting infected in the process. This added hazard to policing has implications for their families. Not only do those families experience divorce and domestic violence at higher rates than other families, now the coronavirus may infect them at high rates. The higher risk for infection also applies to EMTs, nurse aides, and physical therapists who handle people every day, among other similar occupations that involve touching people. Masks and gloves will only go so far in preventing infections when handling closely a lot of others.

However, since most in the service sector of the economy have low incomes they therefore do not have the best of health care, or none that they can afford. The lower paid retail sales clerks, cashiers, restaurant workers and many others mostly earn little and additionally most of these are women.

Essentially, most of the service sector in reference to gender is comprised of women, which is one of the reasons they are paid less. At first, bank tellers were almost all men and working conditions were good for them. These working conditions reversed course when almost all of them who started entering the occupation were women. Now there are a good number of them who are women and some men, both not in ideal conditions after it was mostly women in that occupation.

Many who work in unstable jobs such as commission sales need to be very engaging with others if they are to make sales. Thus, they did a lot of handshaking and worked quite closely with their customers. There are some questions about all this now.

Since many in these service occupations earn low income or now are the long-term unemployed, these workers are more likely to have predisposing conditions of poor health even if they are younger. The elderly, though, are more so in a vulnerable condition as well due to their poorer health because of their age. The predisposing conditions are a result of the relative lack of health insurance, poorer nutrition, unhealthy environments, etc., in contrast to those who are better-off, disproportionately preventing them from accessing health care, especially preventive health care. Thus it is that poor whites and blacks and Latinos (the latter two more likely than whites to be of lower income in comparison and in poorer health consequently) incur more infections and death from the coronavirus. People of color are contracting the virus at a younger age than whites, thus the virus a greater threat to them than to whites.

In other lines of work other than services, many factory workers on the other hand do not interact with a large number of people on a daily, direct basis. Some who work on assembly lines in the meat and poultry industry, still, work shoulder to shoulder all day. Acrylic shields between them are not going to be very practical in the work they do.

There are laboratory workers who focus on what they do which does not involve much interaction with different people other than co-workers. Then there are those who do repair work on automobiles, electronics, etc., and do so basically in their own physical work area. Repair people overall cannot wear gloves in their occupation or be constantly sanitizing what the customers bring to them. Moreover, of those who do wear gloves and face masks in their occupation or elsewhere may very well contaminate themselves when they take them off, if they do so incorrectly. This was not a society of face mask and glove wearers before, so this is novel, as the coronavirus too is called novel.

Some of the most sought-after jobs now are those where an employee is working at home, because of the virus. Even though these positions involve telecommunicating with others, there is not even a modicum sometimes of interaction in physical proximity with coworkers. Interacting in person with others is too often an important factor in working. Moreover, working at home can mean that there are distractions at home as well as other problems.

Nevertheless, those doing relatively solitary work interact with friends and family and are not entirely unlikely to be infected. It must be kept in mind though that their friends and family work mostly in the service sector, interacting with others. Those others may infect them and then they infect the relatively solitary worker friends and family members. The solitary long-haul truck drivers as well as local truck drivers, to begin with, in large measure are not well-off and neither are many of their friends and family. That is already saying that poorer people are more likely to suffer the negative consequences of being infected, what with no or little health insurance and other negative living conditions.

There are others who drive for a living who do interact with a diverse set of customers each day such as taxi drivers, unlike truck drivers. Taxi drivers themselves are more likely to be poor and have friends and family who are poor. These are sociological likelihoods of such categories of people. In other words, in reference to taxi drivers there are not equal numbers of wealthy, middle class, and poor taxi drivers in many quite variegated situations.

It must be said that in a service economy like that of the U.S. there are types of businesses which in pre-coronavirus days relied heavily or entirely on ambience of the particular business. A good example is that of some restaurants which did not even have a take-out window because of the "atmosphere" they were proud to provide. They relied on customers seating inside the place. Then some which did not focus on atmosphere were buffet-type where diners handled the spoons and other items to get food from the trays, which is now not possible as in pre-virus days, but that is what these restaurants relied on.

Now many restaurants will be reconsidering a number of things if they want to stay in business. For one, some will add outdoor tables if they had not already done so, though that may backfire during inclement weather such as rain and cold. For another, they may rearrange the seating inside the restaurant. They probably are not going to have fans, since these blow the aerosols and droplets from the virus throughout the place. All this will be done at their own cost, cutting into their profits.

These situations have been upended and will continue be so for some time, closed as they had to be entirely for many weeks and losing the revenue. Then they only opened at about 25% capacity, then later at 50%, and so forth, which is a losing proposition for many businesses. The restrictions were loosened, then tightened again by some states "opening up" too soon, particularly by those who supported Trump's concern about how his economic system looked. By the time they re-opened and then closed again, the damage had irreversibly been done. Quite a number of establishments have closed for good since they did not have the luxury (cash) to stay afloat until presumably better times in some unforeseeable future, the uncertainty taking its toll on the employees who worked there as well and have been left without immediate prospects for a job elsewhere.

Then again, there were some employers imploring with reluctant employees to return to work. Said employees harbored great anxieties about getting infected. They faced the dilemma of returning to work and possibly getting infected and getting a family member infected (with death as a possibility), or remaining unemployed but perhaps healthy, without money to pay bills and probably being replaced at work. The only question now would be finding work thereafter, an increasingly questionable proposition.

Once it was realized that contagiousness of the virus was high at meat packing plants these businesses were closed. Then Trump classified that industry as essential and basically ordered the re-opening of the plants. The workers were told to return, though some said they would not because of the risk of infection. Acrylics placed between these workers are not practical, and are more so for show and pretensions about concern for workers.

The meat packers had already lost profits before being initially closed down, since restaurants which would have bought their meat were closed for many weeks, not to mention that unemployed consumers did not have much money for expensive meat. Throughout the pandemic it is clear where priorities are, primarily in reference to profit.

When some do not work due to the above reasons about infection, or during strikes, there are what are called scabs who employers readily hire to replace at lower pay the former employees. Scabs without a family can move more readily. Many are younger without other job prospects and are less likely than older workers to become ill with COVID-19. If they live alone they don't have others, in comparison to those who are married and have a family, to transmit the infection. Moreover, their parents and grandparents might live far away.

The undocumented are in precarious situations. They keep a low profile to avoid deportation. They are desperate for income, often sending much of it to their families in their home country. Employers know all this and find it easier to exploit them. A number of the occupations of the undocumented are unsafe, with injuries commonplace but without recourse about such injuries. In various ways they are among the most vulnerable for super-exploitation. Many of them work in conditions which make infection more likely with no social distancing, etc.

In this way society pays less for their services, etc., since the employers unfortunately pay them less. Not many investigate their rates of infection. As is the case with prisoners, many in society are not concerned about the undocumented.

Of those who are told to return to work in virus-risky jobs, many are people of color. Those who work as hair stylists and nail salons and the like are examples of this. (With fewer haircuts perhaps the style of longer hair will return as it perforce had when the salons were closed.) Then some would rather not return at a certain point in time to work, but not have much choice about that such as restaurant workers, particularly servers who earn much of their income in tips, when and if they do earn tips. Sometimes they hope against hope to earn a decent living as they may previously had been doing from tips.

That may not be the case now that many diners would rather order take-out, or worse for restaurant workers, not eat out anymore and instead eat at home, what with the risks of interacting with restaurant workers who may be infected, or with other diners. Food may be prepared by cooks without a mask and even touching the plates, etc. (without gloves, of course, said gloves getting dirty and harboring perhaps more of the virus). The food itself may not be a great problem, since cooked food apparently does not harbor much of the virus. Inspectors, however, generally pay less than a handful of visits to restaurants in any given year, if any.

Something not mentioned often by those in political office seeking to have employees return to work is that their return will end the unemployment compensation payments to those who had been unemployed due to the virus. This is not all that different than the efforts by some to get those receiving government assistance foisted onto a worthless job or training. Countless of the low income employed cannot afford much for food, rent, etc. Employers of the latter jobs sometimes themselves get monetary assistance by the government to hire in dead end jobs those receiving "welfare," with the employer being the main beneficiary of it all.

Of course, for many of these low paid workers there is no day care they can afford. Furthermore, day care centers are now becoming places where the virus spreads, akin to the nursing home situation. Then the parents, grandparents and others would be infected, more seriously so than younger people. All this is in addition to the fact that those who return to work do need some sort of childcare. They were taking care of their own children when schools closed.

It will be interesting to see how schools which had after-school care/programs will fare when schools re-open, since many parents, particularly poor parents, cannot be home for their children right after school and had relied on these centers as a type of childcare place until the parent got home. Nevertheless, after-school programs will be needed now more than ever due to the uncertain hours of the jobs currently available, and the jobs of the future (the contingent type of jobs elaborated here later).

Some colleges are modifying their academic calendars to avoid classroom type of courses during a good part of the winter. The fear is that there may be a resurgence of the coronavirus at that time, as there often is of the flu. Finals would be online. It is not that easy for K-12 schools to do this, since their academic year is much longer overall than that of higher education and runs throughout the winter, except for the two weeks of holidays.

The pent-up economic demands that politicians emphasize will not be that pent-up after all if there is a possibility of death in the process which before the virus had not been factored. Vaccines and treatments alone won't salvage the losses and the lingering uncertainties in society.

There may not be pent up demands for certain things, such as certain forms of recreation. As just one example, bowlers might have to buy their own bowling balls instead of sticking their fingers in balls that others used right before them. If they buy bowling balls it will be at the player's expense, and companies which sell them might profit more than they did before. In addition, renting out used bowling shoes will become a problem. There may not be that many workers at bowling alleys (who are paid little) all the time to sanitize everything, and definitely not a full-time position allotted for just doing that.

No decent analysis is made of why things happen and the meaning of it all and the consequences. The coronavirus will continue to wreak havoc in the meantime, just as terrorism, crime and other maladies continue to do, but the deadly virus is now ever-present in the background of society hereafter in the U.S. and around the world. Very significantly and rather immediately the coronavirus is changing many societies. It is infecting people in this society and throughout the world on a continuous basis, unlike terrorism and even murder which occur intermittently and at discrete moments, according to crime clocks.

Some issues arise in regard to vaccines, treatments and testing. Vaccines such the one for the flu are not entirely successful, with those vaccinated sometimes still coming down with the flu. There are variants of the flu and different vaccines try to address this at certain time intervals, be it annually or otherwise. Moreover, not everyone gets the flu vaccine. Affordable health care that includes vaccination is not what everyone has in his or her pocketbook. Those without resources for the vaccine may become infected with the coronavirus and infect others. Furthermore, even though this is a pandemic, it is not feasible that every person in the world will be vaccinated.

Treatment works for those infected with something that is treatable. They can still get infected again, most likely those who work in the service sector coming across others who are infected. There are people, for example, with gonorrhea who have been infected with it and treated many times. There are those with syphilis likewise who are treated for it successfully yet still may get it at another point in time. It is possible that a person may in time be treated for COVID-19, yet get it again. This same person can instead be vaccinated after treatment, though with the above social problems associated with some vaccinations.

Testing comes with its own problems, so to speak, the most prominent being that the results are good for today, but if infected tomorrow a new test would have to be administered to find that out. Daily testing for the great majority of the population, not to mention all of the population, is surreal and certainly would never be a reality for all the people in the world, except for the wealthy who would opt for that. Moreover, before administration of the test and the results, untold thousands or millions are anxious for the test results in the interim, adding another layer of anxiety in society. In fact, some of the results that indicate a person is positive for it may be incorrect, a false positive. Some of the results are a false negative indicating that a person is not infected when in fact they are and thereby can infect others.

It should go without saying that in the sociological sense, some categories of people will be more likely than others to be vaccinated, to be treated, and to be tested and are thereby privileged. There is no equality across the board on these matters, and this situation is no different than other things in society, such as education, health care, etc.

Chapter 2

Relationships

In sociology there is the concept of the presentation of self. People present themselves to others for particular reasons and purposes. This depends on the situation. There is now a seismic shift in how all of this is being transformed by the coronavirus.

Relationships with others are changing dramatically. For one thing, it needs to be clarified that "social distance" was originally a sociological concept. It was not about keeping six feet of physical distance from others. It was and still pertains to the concept of the level of interaction all people deem they want to maintain in regard to others' racial/ethnic backgrounds. Namely, some people would not want another category of people in the U.S., or they would be OK with a category of people being in the country but not in their region of the country, and so forth for various levels of interaction down to whether for some it is OK with the son or daughter dating those of a certain category but not marrying them. Where there would be no social distance is when parents, for example, would be OK with their son or daughter marrying someone of a certain racial/ethnic category.

Social distance, sociologically speaking, therefore can mean that some don't want those from certain racial/ethnic categories even in the country, whereas on the other hand some are OK with there being no social distance from those of certain racial/ethnic categories. In sum, that is the original sociological definition of what is now being called social distance, before the coronavirus.

Social distance thus in reference to the coronavirus is sociologically incorrect. Social distance is not used as a sociologically meaningful concept at all now in common usage, but only as the physical distance people keep from one another, six feet generally, though originally the insistence was on ten feet instead, whereas others said four feet.

In short, interaction and interpersonal communication have suffered a setback from whatever progress there may have been in society prior to the virus. This is most damaging to race relations, in one sense. Basically, the idea of "sticking to one's own" will likely gain ground in terms of overall relations with others. Those who were uncomfortable already with others of different racial, ethnic and cultural backgrounds will be even more so now that there is a risk of infection, however slight the risk may be. The risk will become the excuse not to interact much with these others now.

In stark contrast to the above, many will find it more incumbent upon themselves to understand more about race relations and therefore those of different backgrounds. That is due to the teachable moments from the protests about police brutality and the greater awareness now that black lives do matter, since before they did not much matter, certainly not in comparison to white lives and/or police lives, etc. The question will be whether all this will lead to greater interaction with each other racially, as would seem to be the case in such circumstances. Then again, as pointed out above, there will also be a reluctance to simply interact with others: a fear of infection will be significantly present for some time. In other words, a tendency to not interact with others because of the coronavirus will vie with a tendency to interact racially with others for a better understanding of others.

Unfortunately, way too many are going to be more reticent in their interactions and relationships with others, including those they know to some significant extent, but this is worse in reference to an increased reticence in their interactions with those they do not know. Those who were shy will feel vindicated about being shy. Those who were proud of being able to make friends with others that easily will perhaps now feel a letdown in not being as able to befriend as they did before, lest they get infected and thereby infect others also.

Moreover, in the 1960s those who grew up during the "summer of love" will think about that as quite nostalgic, quaint even, and unfortunately relegated to the mists of time. A lot of the meaning of togetherness is becoming lost now. Essentially, many will perceive others as suspect carriers of the contagious disease.

This is of pertinence in a great many situations. For example, those who did not want to hand out a dollar to a homeless person will be less inclined now to do so, lest there be some accidental touching involved and possibly infection, or even the very breathing of the homeless spreading droplets and possibly infection. Of course the homeless will think the same of the person handing him or her a dollar bill, a possibly contaminated dollar bill at that, but the homeless will have less choice about it, as in general those not well off do not have many choices. The circumstances of the homeless will become more grim than they already were in our society. Even soup kitchens in communities may now become suspect by the participants, particularly by some who volunteered.

The very handshake which had been a staple of relationships, whether for business or personal reasons throughout millennia, is going now in the direction of the extinct dodo bird. Countless occupations rely on the handshake as a way of communicating a number of positive things, whether in sales, agency work, or most any kind of employment. A handshake has become unlikely for fear of contracting the contagious virus.

There were, of course, those who were proud of their hearty handshake. Then there were those who were insecure in their dead fish type of handshake. Both types will now also reconsider themselves, generally the former in a negative way and the latter in a positive way. The lack of a handshake modifies relationships as does the lack of hugging for the huggers and the lack of a smile for the masked.

Those who risk getting infected and are perhaps more concerned about consummating a sale may wind up infecting not only themselves but others, which would not be a positive outcome from earning a commission from that sale, or finalizing a contract, etc., particularly if a family member dies from the infection. Greetings now will settle for a tilt of the head, elbow bumps, or something else in our society which was not at all that quite common before the coronavirus.

There are cultural variants throughout the world for greeting others, but a firm handshake had been central particularly in Western society. For example, before the virus the handshake was perceived as the norm while an elbow bump would have been considered an oddity. The awkward elbow bump in a matter of weeks became normalized to a significant extent in our own society, though not all that desirable yet as a norm to replace the handshake. Shaking hands, however, is now perceived as doing so at one's peril.

Alongside the greeting of one another with a handshake was a smile or what would pass for a smile. With face masks smiles are not that visible, though other parts of the face which change when one smiles can be glimpsed with a greater attentiveness to the rest of the face. Some intercom recordings in stores stated that customers practice "social distancing" but that they could still acknowledge each other with a smile were incongruous with said customers wearing a face mask. The face mask, of course, covered not only the mouth used for smiling, it also was supposed to cover the nose and go over the chin, which is quite an area of the face in addition to the mouth.

Those who smiled a lot or frowned a lot now have second thoughts about how to express themselves when wearing a face mask. The phrase "masking their real selves" takes on a whole new meaning. Some were very proud of their smile, perhaps because people said they had a very nice smile, or because they felt very happy in smiling at others, or simply because they had very good teeth to show. The opposite of all this may have been the case for those who did not smile that often.

The importance of the mask is self-explanatory in mitigating the spread of the virus and perhaps became more vital than the act of smiling, since not everyone before was smiling at each other anyway. Even though many were insincere and gave a fake smile before when involved in social interaction with each other such as with fellow employees and/or with customers, in the more meaningful and personal relationships smiling was very desirable with friends and family nonetheless. With a mask it becomes more difficult to perceive smiles and therefore perceive the nuances of everyday interactions with others. However, there are now masks which are transparent where the mouth is and therefore smiles can be seen as they were before, as an important part of one's expression. There are not that many of those types of face masks yet and perhaps will not catch on. Furthermore, some masks are emblazoned with slogans, artwork, and other forms of expression. Some wear the larger bandanas as facial coverings, which therefore cover the neck, but masks are more common than bandanas.

One situation where smiling was very meaningful was in dating, particularly when the desire to date someone obviously was preceded sometimes with a warm smile. Now when meeting someone dateable, with both persons wearing a mask, that conveyance of warmth and desire became a little bit more of a problem, a song and dance, so to speak, and more urgent. What would pass for a nice smile before now had to be amplified with a bigger smile which would therefore show other parts (muscles) of the face in order to convey that a person was definitely smiling.

Some misunderstandings are inevitable under these circumstances as to whether a person wanted or didn't want to pursue an acquaintanceship after just having met. For example, before the virus the lack of reciprocating a smile would nip in the bud any furtherance of acquaintanceship. Again, nonverbal communication within a culture is not all that difficult to "read" or determine, but sometimes it is. Very often it is definitely too difficult to "read" in cross-cultural communication/ interaction.

It needs to be added that although many in our society now use facial masks, this has long been the case in some cultures such as in certain Islamic societies. In Afghanistan many women are covered from head to toe, though in other Islamic societies not the entire body is covered while still in others only a small veil or no veil is requisite. In case some people think that Islamic women are the only ones veiled, among Christians themselves a veil on top of the head was expected among Catholic women while at mass in recent history. When photographs are seen of Jackie Kennedy at the funeral of her assassinated husband, she is wearing a laced black veil covering her entire head and neck.

One of the very reasons for veiling in Islam and one which many Islamic women believe is that a woman should be perceived for what she is and does in society and therefore for her capacities, which do not include being a sex object as many women are in Western societies. In the U.S.

quite often women are seen as a sex object by men and not for what women as persons are and do and their capacities as respected professionals, for example. Sexual assaults of women in the military occur at a higher rate than in society in general, regardless of their capacities in the military.

The eyes of many will drift even more than they do now to looking at others' eyes since the mouth can't be seen due to masking. The eyes communicate much. Even some who wear sunglasses, such as police and security people, do so in order that others will not read their eyes, but not necessarily because of the sun's glare. Skills at reading eyes will develop rapidly. Obviating all this are persons who wear sunglasses and a mask, in essence nullifying all facial expressions. Of interest is seeing how people react to these persons.

Those who hugged a lot and those who did not hug much will reconsider their circumstances, in light of the coronavirus, in projecting their real selves. Namely those who were "huggers" may feel at a disadvantage without the hugging, now with the possibility of infection or infecting others, particularly if they or others are asymptomatic. Perhaps they may feel they have lost an intrinsic part of themselves in being unable to hug others. When and if they do hug others, those hugged may feel awkward or uncomfortable about the encounter in contrast to before.

On the other hand, those (the non-huggers) who felt uncomfortable about hugging may feel vindicated. Others are also feeling vindicated such as those who were germophobic or were paranoid about being contaminated with something or other, not only by people who may be infected but also by touching surfaces of all types as well (some surfaces harbor the virus for a longer or shorter period of time). If the latter resort to wearing gloves, they may be picking up more of the virus on the glove and then contaminating themselves if they are not careful about taking the gloves off; ditto about those not careful when taking off a mask which may harbor contaminated droplets.

Hugging may be expected and desirable while on a date, though it may not occur on a first date. Hugging conflicts with the precept of keeping a distance from others (the distancing an impossibility for dates riding in a car and certainly the distancing of six feet is a contradiction in terms of what a date is all about). Social distancing is not what couples want while dating. In an instance when neither of the two are wearing masks and are only a foot or so away from each other in a car or in a restaurant, talking with each other may result in infecting the other, particularly when they do not know each other well at that point. This may dictate talking at a low volume at that close of a distance, because even at greater distances loud talkers spew out more aerosols and droplets which reach others.

Passing a contagion to another when hugging, which occurs in very close interaction, can occur whether in dating or in greeting friends. The same applies for simply holding hands on a date, obviously. Perhaps worst of all in a way is kissing in the passing of a contagion. Thus it is that kissing on the first date will for many be deferred to much later on for those who do not know each other very well, even though they may definitely want to know each other as soon and as well as possible. There is even what many refer to as love at first sight (or at least second sight sometimes) and such a person who is falling in love may not want to delay kissing and hugging for too long. At some point the couple may just chuck all reservations about kissing by the wayside.

In a word, kissing on dates will become quite more conditional than what it may have been before. Even if a couple, or one of the couple, believes that they should get to know each other better, nothing can guarantee that the person(s) are free of the virus without some documentation of it. Paperwork for dating would take on a whole new meaning at that juncture. Dating would certainly become quite awkward if couples were very determined to have documentation of testing on hand before much or any physical contact. Still, that would clearly not guarantee that the person presenting it did not get infected since the dated testing on the paperwork.

Now the dating process will be reconsidered. As a matter of fact, those dating may experience new anxieties, while those not dating may be glad they are not doing so at that point in time. When they start or re-start dating that is another matter. Much of this was articulated to some extent about AIDS when it came along a few decades ago. Even then many who dated had thrown caution to the wind, with some serious consequences. The same applies to other sexually transmitted illnesses. The common refrain about AIDS and STIs that these are not spread through casual interactions does not apply to the coronavirus. In case of this virus, the higher volume talking produces more air droplets nearby and the even smaller aerosols up to some distances. Moreover, mere touching may be enough to infect someone else with the coronavirus.

In fact, Britain at a point in 2020 added to their restrictions about the coronavirus by making it illegal to engage in sex with someone outside a person's household. It would presumably include those who are having affairs. It remains to be seen how this plays out in time. This is exactly, though, what very intimate interactions with those a person does not know well would entail, especially if the person is asymptomatic. Infecting a person with an STI is one thing, now there is this exponentially increasing virus contamination from perhaps a mere touch, or even breathing, by someone. Some today even assault someone by coughing on him or her on purpose.

The coronavirus infections are not confined, though, to a subset of society, but occur throughout much of American society and the world without respect to age, dating patterns, etc. The virus is transmitted much more easily and casually than STDs from one person to another, though sexual interactions pose still an additional avenue of transmission from touching alone. Moreover, death from COVID-19 comes about. if and when it does, much more swiftly, within a matter of weeks than it does from AIDS and syphilis when these STDs are left untreated. Most recover from the coronavirus infection, though, which cannot be said for infections from the above two STDs if left untreated, which simply progress in time with deleterious consequences.

Not only that, a person may be infected by the coronavirus after he or she starts dating. If the couple were to be tested for the virus, the results may be negative but one of them or both may be infected later on in the relationship by someone else and in turn infect the dating partner. It almost becomes a question of how often they want to test or produce a health certificate of some sort and documentation of testing, which may not be feasible or affordable on a daily or weekly basis.

This means that there will be discrimination against some categories of people by much of society. This particular type of discrimination may develop as to who will be chosen for dating partners and even who people eventually will marry. Parents often ask their son or daughter about the intentions of those they date, concerned as they are about the array of choices of their son or daughter for a possible marriage partner and welcoming this person into the fold of the family. Now the concern is furthermore possibly a matter of death (though an outside possibility) for a member of the family. Parents may now insist on testing for the virus for the dating partner of their son or daughter. Some parents will want to see the documentation of such testing and the results, again the test good only for now and not predictive about infection in the future, particularly the near future.

Even the most attractive in society will harbor doubts about the frequency of dating others and about the number of others attracted to them. More loneliness may be in the cards for those seeking relationships, what with the uncertainties about other people. Desperation may very well become more of a reality for many who date and in particular for those who are seriously looking for someone to marry.

The personal ads and dating services will attempt to adapt in ways perhaps currently unforeseen. Some of them already had asked for documentation about some things. Possibly a brisk business may develop in forged test results and documents, as is the case in forged or fake social security cards/numbers sold on the street to some applicants for certain types of employment.

There is a possibility that another result will be street prostitutes more actively seeking their clients (johns), since many prostitutes are in economic straits and cannot be concerned about medical or other matters very much. These johns, though they may get desperate for sex from them, may be fearful of contracting the coronavirus since it is more easily transmitted than STIs. The mere acts of touching and talking with another can trigger an infection if the prostitute is contagious. Still, much of prostitution involves organized crime, and the latter is ruthless about its business dealings. Even the discreet drug transactions of organized crime will more easily result in infection from those who are contagious. Prostitution and illegal drugs often coincide.

For those who are married a cascade of relationship problems will arise from extensive unemployment from a job disappearing altogether or even merely the lower income from hours cut from a job. Part time work may be all that is available, the new reality.

It is not only domestic violence from these tensions that will arise. The incidence of divorce increases under these circumstances, which is not to say it definitely will in all marriages encountering financial problems. In turn this can affect children in some ways often negatively, but sometimes positively when there was family violence before the divorce. Divorce may be positive for children in a household of domestic violence. If divorce does not occur as an outcome of layoffs, there may be more conflict in that intact family about unpaid bills, etc.

The question may devolve into that of counseling for conflict-ridden marriages. Since counselors and therapists practiced telemedicine before the coronavirus, this will now increase, in comparison with the previous face-to-face sessions. Telemed counseling with children of divorcing parents, or for that matter any children, will be quite a problem. Effectiveness will be a challenge for various clients in an increasingly telemed world. Whatever the effectiveness, insurance companies are increasingly less interested now in covering telemed and telehealth virtual sessions, and have made the process more onerous therefore by having more authorizations needed for virtual appointments.

Those majoring in counseling might begin to harbor second thoughts about the merits of virtual therapy. Not the least of concerns is the lesser pay for counseling when it is telemed. This bears a similarity to the lower pay for instructors of online courses and obviously the lower cost of online courses as well. Patients/clients more than likely also will want to pay less for telemed than the face-to-face.

Whenever in-person sessions do occur, therapists and counselors may now demand documentation that a person has been tested for the virus. Having a mask on and being six feet away are not factors in very effective counseling. Counselors obviously will check the temperature of their clients as dentists and so many other professionals now do, which they did not do before the virus. The ubiquitous touchless thermometers are only matched by the proliferation of a touchless world. Masks and gloves will make for less effective communication and all in all an increasingly awkward situation. However, those in other jobs such as EMTs and the police do not have the luxury of asking others for health documentations and a touchless approach in their work.

In relation to the coronavirus, we already have in society some problem people engaged in TV counseling. Dr. Phil, whose licensure has been questioned to practice counseling, was incensed that the economy was closed and claimed that simultaneously there were more deaths from other causes than the virus. He said that 360,000 died yearly from drowning in swimming pools, which is ridiculous.

Oprah promoted him after he was on her show, as she is wont to do with those she likes, and now we have his show. His publicity is what made it possible to tout the false 360,000 dead. That's not all. He also made a false equivalence to the virus in even mentioning other types of deaths. Those other deaths are not contagious, though, as the coronavirus is. He in fact is instead supposed to focus on relationships. Yet it is really impossible for anyone to claim to accomplish much of anything in a TV show of less than an hour (commercials included, which are the main thing about the show, the sponsors for people to go out and buy their wares). That is not to mention that there is something untoward of so-called therapy with millions of voyeurs watching. Any social scientist will immediately state that this will contort what are supposed to be the candid dynamics of family members on those couches.

Overall, the actual question is more simple, a crass one: it is a matter of whether to profiteer from opening an economy soon vs deaths from the virus. The cold economic calculations have been laid bare for everyone to now see regarding relationships and realize what society is about. It is not about health concerns. In case anyone did not get the point, it was clarified by Texas Lt. Governor Patrick, a former rightwing radio host, who became apoplectic in his exclamation that the markets needed to be open even if it meant that some people die.

Patrick only illustrates, as do Trump and others, their anxiety over the economic system, while they shed crocodile tears over deaths. Patrick said he wanted to save the economy for his offspring, who happen to be white, even if people died from the virus. Not surprisingly in a similar way, the U.S. military stated or implied during the Vietnam War that it became necessary to destroy towns there in order to save them. Patrick is failing on both counts: the economy is collapsing and people are dying.

What Patrick did not say is that the economy has been one geared to benefit whites and that the coronavirus affects blacks and Latinos more than whites due to historically racist socioeconomic factors. Black and Latino lives have been considered more expendable. Malcolm X was well known for indicating that the white man appears to speak for the black man, or that the master's interests were supposedly those of the slave. As he put it, some slaves believed that to the point of the house slave putting out a fire engulfing the master's house. This is familiar in the situation of some black police officers following the racist ethos of police departments, even if it costs black suspects their lives.

The corollary today to relationships within those of a racial category, briefly, is that some blacks are thus referred to as oreos, blacks on the outside but white on the inside. Said Latinos are referred to as coconuts, brown on the outside but white on the inside (also referred to as vendidos among the Spanish speaking: sellouts). Such blacks and Latinos are not going to accept (because they get the same messages much of society gets) that it is the socioeconomic conditions they find themselves in which lead to higher rates of infections and deaths, or that lead to much of anything else such as lower levels of education, of health, of jobs, etc. Even whites in the U.S. in the spring and summer of 2020 now realized, much more than before the virus, that racism was and is systemic, including in police departments and elsewhere throughout society, and that it is not a case of bad apples or individuals who are problem people.

One of the situations where racist interactions were made public other than the above was by a reference to Karens. Although the origin of the term is unclear, a Karen in 2020 came to be the appellation to white women (and some white men) whose racism in various places, such as at stores, parks, and elsewhere was recorded on cell phones. These recordings became viral on the internet.

The corporate peculiarity of Patrick in Texas against workers came to light when Congressional Senator Ted Cruz of the same state exclaimed that oil prices had collapsed. He said one main reason for that is because the "truck" in the driveway is not moving due to stay-at-home policies. He also referred to planes not using oil because they are not flying. He was exasperated that all this would lead to millions of jobs lost. Again, he like many others, is not concerned about workers but is concerned about airlines, gas stations, and other related corporations and their profits.

Cruz, Patrick, and Trump have never concerned themselves with the welfare, pay, and rights of workers. They are staunchly anti-union, against teachers' unions and others. The worker is only useful to them in buying stuff for the profit of the corporations. Workers and their relationships with their families primarily matter to the corporate entities to the extent that some can die, are expendable, and the corporation will immediately go on to the next applicant in line for the job.

At the workplace and elsewhere the coronavirus can be asymptomatic and one may have no idea of being infected yet will be infecting others in his or her relationships. The symptoms moreover are varied. A fever does not necessarily mean infection with this virus, though a fever now may be enough to send people to testing. The fever may mean they will not be provided with a service of some sort, such as when he or she goes in for dental work. Extensive testing for the virus is not feasible publicly nor is it all that privately affordable.

Basically, the choices for relationships may narrow substantially regardless whether there is a vaccine, treatment and extensive testing. The very testing itself brings about anxieties as most any testing does. The anxieties are relieved briefly only for the time being until the next test. By the time medical advances come about much of society will have become leery of others much more so than before. That certainly is not conducive to bringing society together in a positive way, though it was not together all that much before the virus and in fact there was plenty of polarization, discrimination, racism, and so forth already. Risk aversiveness against others may gain ground at the expense of social cohesiveness and working together.

Those who seek relationships with others are likely now consulting other cultures and seeing what they can apply and learn from them about dating, friendships, etc. There is much variation among cultures. Even within the U.S. there are some who blow a kiss to another person instead of physically kissing that person on the cheek. That was looked down upon by others before the coronavirus as a way of showing affection, akin to a pre-virus detesting of elbow bumps and tilting of heads, both now acceptable norms, to acknowledge another instead of shaking hands.

Some of the anxieties may stem from younger people who may be asymptomatic and thus afraid that they may be transmitting the virus to their older family members. On the other hand, the older family members may also fear possible transmission from younger people (such as older teachers fearing that from their young students) and in particular from younger family members. The immune systems of the older are more compromised than those of the younger and therefore they die at greater rates from the infection by the virus. A possible exception is that older people who can afford to have better health care can still overcome problems sometimes because their immune systems and general health are better when they have been tended to in accordance with their financial ability to do so.

There are occasions when it is expected that the elderly come together with the younger, such as at Thanksgiving. This now poses some questions. Since the younger may infect the older, both the younger and older will reconsider how close they will be at the dinner table. Even if not at the dinner table, they still interact with each before and after the dinner. Around the table all are elbow to elbow. To keep six feet from each other means only about two diners around a large table. These reunions mostly involve more than two people who come together for Thanksgiving, as has been the case up until now. Three or four shifts at the table defeats the purpose of all socializing around the table on this holiday.

It remains to be seen how the relationships change from the younger in regard to their elderly aunts, uncles and grandparents. It is possible that someone whose age is in the twenties yet asymptomatic of the virus may become less inclined to get too close to the grandparent out of concern from the younger one of possibly infecting the grandparent. The younger person might have been recently interacting with others rather closely and therefore not sure if he or she got infected, short of being tested.

Obviously when the grandparent is ill with something, the younger person will now likely refrain from interacting with the grandparent. That is a very high likelihood given that formally no one has been allowed inside nursing homes lately to interact in person with the residents other than staff, with precautions. The message is clear for family members, particularly the younger family members.

Perhaps a decent meal with a small family gathering is in the offing now, instead of turkeys with all the trimmings for large numbers of people (the decent meal and smaller gathering would be a relief for the women who generally do the unthankful work of cooking for large numbers, while too many men generally sit around the TV watching football games, often with beers in hand). The same applies to Christmas and other holidays/reunions.

If these occasions for gatherings become a moot point, many may come to realize that there were after all ulterior motives by some in society to emphasize some holidays, such as Christmas. Namely, profit-hungry entities led us to think that people wanted others to buy presents for them, "it's better to give than to receive," for the corporations' profits that is. Consumerism predominates, so far. The same might be said about Valentine's Day, for example. Flower shops and restaurants make profits from that holiday.

Just being together for such holidays was not enough before, but now may be. Moreover, the process of being together might change qualitatively, but also quantitatively. This means money won't be spent to buy that many presents. The madness might subside of Black Friday after Thanksgiving, wherein corporations gauge if they are going to be in the black for the year from profits (instead of in the red), hence the name.

The spending associated with these holidays may become unsustainable anyway due to the unemployment from the coronavirus upending the economy as well as from efforts to mitigate the risk of infection. On the other hand, the togetherness may become more significant, particularly in smaller family gatherings than in the huge gatherings of those related and unrelated or even unknown to each other.

Furthermore, with the togetherness being more meaningful, all this might eliminate the conflicts that arise during these and other larger gatherings/ holidays.

Also clear is that some gatherings remind people of the very relationships they have with others, particularly if they are strained relationships. Perceived shortcomings in those relationships contribute to the occurrence of suicides. The social patterns of suicides are clearly evident in terms of its demographics, time frames, history, cultures, gender, and so forth. Much of the distress is social in the sense that when workers are let go in large numbers as they have been due to the virus then those in the category of the unemployed may second guess themselves. They might ponder why the boss let them go instead of someone else, particularly when a corporation claims that it is downsizing.

The ones still working are not out of the woods as far as distress is concerned, because now there is speed up. This is when those who remain are expected to do more work, generally the work of the downsized employee. The stress results from the fear of being let go themselves if and when they do not produce as expected, mind you without the boss paying for the speed up, or not paid much for doing the work of the one let go. There is the army of the unemployed waiting outside the employer's door to replace employees who are let go.

The remaining work force has bills to pay, etc., and does almost whatever the boss demands in order to stay in the good graces of the boss. They become more malleable. Workers are now even sleeping less, concerned as they are about their dire circumstances overall and the stress of the working conditions. Some are made to work longer hours by the boss. That is something not found in much of Europe. Yet pay has not increased accordingly, nor commensurate with speed up here. In some European countries employees instead work thirty-some hours per week on average while they receive relatively free health care, free college, free day care, and so forth.

There is not much of a meaningful and comprehensive societal safety net for those unemployed here as is the case in various European and other societies. The employee here does for the employer, without the latter reciprocating much, particularly in the form of paying taxes for societal purposes. Corporations now pay the lowest taxes than they did in the 1950s. The apprehensiveness of workers is palpable and exemplified in higher rates of crime and other problems in this particular society.

Poor whites and people of color are more so affected by the social misery concomitant with this virus than the better-off and whites in general. Not much is written about this in the U.S. because it rips open the scab of massive inequality for all to see. There is less inequality in European and other countries where higher education and health care, for example, are provided for and easily afforded for practically everyone. Such countries have a higher life expectancy and other social indicators are better than here. This is not to say that people from here go there, but that positive circumstances be made a reality here.

When it comes to discrimination leading to inequality, there appears to be a type of discrimination that may increase more substantially than what is now the case. Namely, since New York state, particularly the city, has had a disproportionate number of COVID-19 cases and deaths in comparison to other states and cities, many people elsewhere may very well come to feel uncomfortable around New Yorkers. The same applies to discrimination against those from New Orleans and other "hotspots" as they have come to be called. Already that has been the case officially in that those from Louisiana going to another state have been required to quarantine themselves. Of course, the location of "hotspots" change as we speak, with Texas becoming a more significant one in many ways than others were, especially after a hasty "re-opening."

The spike in infections changes, such that now there is a significant increase in cases in rural areas and small towns, the very areas that many are going to when they flee the larger cities, such as New York City. Some of those who flee and look for homes in rural areas and towns gratuitously mention they are also fleeing conflict in the city, which is code for the racial protests lately. Wouldn't you know it, though, those fleeing are whites who more likely can work remotely from their home, which is to say those who have a higher income than others.

This gives the former concept of white flight from the cities a new meaning, a new wrinkle, now in reference to the virus. Before it was just racial reasons. Apparently, these whites may not have supported the protests in the first place, but fleeing to a location that is spiking in infections may not be the most rational choice. They may realize the mistake when it is too late, when they have already bought a house in the new locale.

Many people cannot afford to move, especially if they do not have a decent job waiting for them upon arrival. Therefore, the more virus-laden places might lose some population from those who are better-off and can afford to be more mobile. Those in more unstable circumstances, especially those with a family in tow, will resent that they do not have the wherewithal to go anywhere and that they are stuck in fluctuating and bleak job prospects as well as more coronavirus infections therein, and deaths. That does not make for happy residents of a city or state, venting their frustrations on others. Before, there were many who did resent the dire situation they found themselves in where they were living. Now added to the mix is still more economic turbulence, along with new health anxieties.

Still another way that a new form of discrimination will materialize perhaps is in the reluctance of people to vacation not only in The Big Apple, but also in the states of Washington, Louisiana, and New Jersey. Louisiana is promoted as a sportsman's paradise (their wording by the state), and perhaps in that relatively solitary activity of being a sportsman that will be fine. Strolling through a crowded French Quarter in New Orleans is another matter. Some will research where the "hotspots" for the virus are or were and plan vacations avoiding them.

For vacations perhaps the previously crowded Yellowstone National Park will be avoided in favor of less crowded national parks and other attractions. Then again, given the job situation, the money likely won't be there for vacations, maybe not even for crowded nearby theme parks for the family, regardless of how much employees need vacations for a respite, especially a respite from employment where one may be stressed out but still cling to that one available job. It is rather obvious that there is a probability that Italy, Spain and China will be avoided as well as other international destinations. Europeans in the summer of 2020 essentially banned travel from the U.S., in effect banning vacations and other trips to the U.S. lest the Europeans return with the virus. Of course, one could quarantine, but why go through all that rigamarole, per the European frame of mind.

Many cities will suffer financially from the lost revenue from convention attendees, since many conventions are now slated to be virtual instead of in a conference hall. The personal interaction with colleagues will decline. Nurturing these professional contacts has been important in the furtherance of their careers. Talking with each other via a screen is just not the same. To put it simply, much of the excitement outside the conference halls will be lost, the fun of it if you will. Dour relationships with colleagues may result, even if slightly more so than previously.

Even such excitement as that of spring break in college will be reconsidered. Spring breakers will not be as brash as some of those were in spring 2020 who taunted the risk of virus infections, only to sometimes get infected and apologize. Conventions and spring breaks are only some of the perks some people had. Likewise, cruises on ships are not lauded much anymore except by the teetering cruise lines themselves. Being stranded in an ocean or a port would not be the wonderful highlight of one's vacation.

Of course, not only have cruise lines cratered, airlines have already lost a lot of revenue. For the reasons above and others, they are bound to lose even more in time. Whatever excitement there was in flying somewhere will sputter. Flights have already been cut to some destinations. Airlines will dread the consequences financially of a passenger sneezing or coughing, regardless of the actual reason for the passenger doing so, and previously doing so was more likely for relatively innocuous reasons than may be deemed today. It would be no surprise that the violence during flights will increase, as it already had been before the pandemic, from the frustrations of passengers, this while 30,000 feet up in the air and no way to escape what ensues.

The reason for more coronavirus cases from New York, however, has to do with it being the largest city in the congested Northeast in addition to it being a primary disembarkation point for those from Europe and elsewhere, as it was even from the days of immigrants arriving in Ellis Island. The situation in Louisiana, though, is basically a result of the higher rates of the virus spreading as a result of the Mardi Gras close-quarter celebrations. There are reasons for high rates of infection elsewhere. It is not a matter of something inherently bad about people there.

Then again, discrimination to an extent might be experienced by Italians and Spaniards coming to the U.S. Not many people from Wuhan in China would be glad to state that they are from there. With designations of "hotspots" throughout the country, those from there may experience perhaps some discrimination should they mention they are from those locales.

There already has been another type of abhorrence in society. That refers to the now commonly known "lockdowns" which levels of government such as states and cities have imposed. Many no longer see this as mitigation of the spread of the virus. Much of the despising of the government originates from those who want to do what they want, including historically those with racist intentions. Those demonstrating with guns at some state houses were in fact praised by Trump as fine people. They protested to "open up" the state economies (businesses), which really was exactly what Trump sought. They acted as his proxies. He was anxious about any collapse of his vested interest in the economic system, regardless of whoever got infected in the process.

This despising of the government has been the case in the South in particular, recalling the long history of segregation there. Namely, even a governor of Texas, Rick Perry, wrote a book titled Fed Up, indicating that supposedly all Texans were fed up with the federal government, when in fact the modern history of Texas was one of efforts to defy integration of schools in order to maintain segregation. George W. Bush himself revealed he was of that frame of mind about government during a debate as a candidate for president, and at other times, when he stated that his opponent wanted to treat Social Security as if it was a government program (which it is). Governor Wallace of Alabama famously proclaimed "segregation now and forever" during the days of the federal government forcing desegregation there. These anti-government leaders were of the same cloth as the "open the state" protestors. These protestors were mostly white men. In the relationships of the South, racism has figured as a prominent fixture of society.

In a word, the former Confederacy is instead referred to by white southerners as being about states' rights. Yet the very leaders of the Confederacy at the time emphasized it was about slavery. Today it is not about maintaining slavery in the South but about maintaining segregation. Some schools in Houston today are 98% black and Latino. Then there are some which are predominantly white. That applies as well to some schools in the North.

The idea of freeing up and opening up the states, throughout the country and not just in the South, so that some can do what they want is more sinister in its origins and historical backgrounds than appears at first glance. This can easily be gauged today by looking at the type of office holders and their followers who first agitated for "freeing" the states. It would do well to see who they are. To them the coronavirus is an afterthought.

Chapter 3

Education

Higher education and K-12 in the U.S. went online when schools were closed to mitigate the spread of the virus. At first glance this appears as a solution, but it only further exemplified the inequalities in society. For one thing, online higher education and online degrees in particular are considered second-rate by employers in comparison to classroom education and degrees. Discussion and other vital aspects of a college education are rather nonexistent in any meaningful way in the online versions of courses.

Undoubtedly those getting a degree in classroom types of education were more so white, since they were more likely to afford that type of education, a better quality education. The elite universities are disproportionately white and of the classroom type, though even some of these have incorporated a few online courses and even degrees with students enrolled in them for the recognition on paper by these enrollees of getting some sort of education from the elite universities, without much of the better quality of the classroom type in those universities where their white brethren are seated.

The few online degrees from some elite universities are the gate that keeps poorer whites and those of color from their classroom type of education, the more valued type. Even white K-12 "academies" were created to circumvent whites seating next to blacks in schools during and because of desegregation. Additionally, when whites could no longer keep those of color from attending school together, other approaches were utilized.

An example of this was shunting those of color into second-class vocational education classes, which kept them from the college bound classes whites attended in the very same school building. Education supposedly leads to independent and critical thinking, which most places of employment do not welcome (certainly not from uppity students of color) and which vocational education does not foster. It has never been, and still to this day is not, that whites in high school predominate in vocational classes while those of color predominate in college bound classes, even after 70 years of vocational education. Indeed, that would be an anomaly. White parents would not allow anything like that. Inequality, again, manifests itself throughout education and society, including in health care.

Furthermore, there was a scramble to administer the college entrance exams online in 2020, but it became questionable in the sense that fraud is more likely in those formats. Therefore, the idea was to scrap such exams for high school graduates for the fall, though some colleges and the testing services have tried to continue the entrance exams in some guise. Hundreds of universities, including major ones, had anyway stopped using them before, relying on GPA and other factors as criteria for admission. The very future of these entrance exams is in question. The pandemic created a situation to make it possible to question those exams. The formal entrance exams were discriminatory to Latinos and blacks, and they would be among the first to say good riddance to the exams.

With the upcoming de-emphasizing of college entrance exams and the re-emphasizing of GPA and other factors for admission to college, this will become an increased source of stress for some teachers, with parents seeking grade inflation (or worse) in order to get their son or daughter in certain universities. Recent media accounts as well as past history have already uncovered the efforts of the upper class to circumvent entrance exams and bribe or intimidate people associated with colleges to get their sons and daughters admitted to elite universities.

In a word the better-off and mostly white students demand and get the attention of the professor in the classroom and the benefits of the classroom while the less well-off are more likely to attend the second-rate online colleges and get degrees from these. That by itself says a lot about who can afford a better education.

Thus another impact of the coronavirus already is the increase in online higher education overall, which is the more devalued type, at first for all in the beginning of widespread infection in the U.S. soon after spring break 2020, but in time such type of education will be the reality still more so for some but not for others. Online education is being normalized for a large number of students. Not the least of reasons for this was that the high unemployment levels due to the closing of a multitude of nonessential places resulted in unemployed parents realizing they cannot afford anymore whatever classroom type of higher education their sons and daughters were attending, of those who attended these. Many such students are now dropping out of college altogether for the upcoming academic year or are enrolling in the less expensive online type.

Moreover, students who became more financially strapped during the pandemic started to look for jobs, which now were more scarce, to help pay for higher education, if they were to continue in higher education. If they temporarily discontinue their higher education this ensures that graduation will be delayed when and if they do graduate. All these matters of delay and questions about graduation do not affect the better-off white students. The social changes wrought in colleges in the spring of 2020 or at any other time because of the virus affects some more negatively, leaving them behind, and the inequality becomes further entrenched. Moreover, all this as well assumes that in the new online classes everyone has a good computer and internet service. That assumption is incorrect for many in the lower income families.

In the fall of 2020 some elite universities will stagger the education they offer. This means that the classroom type of education will be offered to some but not others in certain semesters or points in time due to the coronavirus. For example, seniors will be more likely to be called back to the classroom courses while perhaps sophomores may not. Those not called back for courses, say, in the fall, may be called back in the spring. Briefly, this burdens the few less well-off students when they are not called back for some semesters because this delays their graduation.

The less well-off cannot afford to delay their education, and in fact might wind up working in the off semester as a way to deal with the situation. They cannot afford to just sit at home in the interim. What is clear is that when students do not attend a semester for whatever reason they are less likely to graduate because of complications from doing so.

They often drop out entirely. The better off-have the means to wait out graduation.

Not only that, when prospective students who are not well-off get wind of these delays, they may very well lose interest in attending some of these universities even though they have a greater need to get the best education. They will go with their second or third choices instead.

Some of the wealthier universities will be testing their students for the virus every few days, while the great majority of Americans cannot be tested on a regular basis, and moreover wait many days or worse to see the results. Most cannot afford to pay for testing and therefore do not get tested, while they may be infectious.

Colleges in general now face a financial dilemma as well. On the one hand, if they open, the education they provide as it was before in the classroom may not get many students in the classroom. Now there are concerns of the institutions for social distancing as well as concerns of students and their families of contracting the virus. Consequently, that means less tuition revenue. If and when they go with some variation of the classroom scenario, colleges in the fall face a probable decline in attendance at football games also for the above reasons, with the optics and the reality of that not looking great for college football, be it that particular college or college football overall. Many colleges are going to play only conference games, if that.

On the other hand, if colleges go with more online type of courses they face a decline in tuition revenue. Online education costs less in tuition since there is no overhead of the classroom type, given the classroom utility costs, maintenance, costs for offices for professors, and so forth. Nevertheless, in the online scenario students and their parents may come to realize that maybe they do not need to be paying the higher tuition of the classroom type, regardless of the fact that the online type is generally inferior in a number of ways. The students and parents may realize that being a graduate of a particular college is more important regardless of how they became a graduate of that college, whether from online or classroom courses.

Already as a result of much of the above there are an increasing number of institutions of higher education that are closing permanently primarily as an outcome of the pandemic's ramifications. That is not much different than businesses such as restaurants and others which closed down completely from the ramifications.

However, another significant question about the classroom courses has sequenced. Namely, if their college football programs are essentially scrapped, that means less revenue for their other sports as well, or simply less total money for the college or university. Even with the first scenarios above of some or much of the classroom type courses or the second scenario of more online courses, another realization occurs. Simply put, the student athletes will conclude, as many had even before the coronavirus, that their playing football brings in revenue for the institution but they do not get any portion of said revenue. The athletes play for free, have less time to study, and some get injured while the college pockets the money/profits. The injuries of the players may be long term.

Another example of economic inequality in education was seen in the insistence by landlords and others that students pay for the remainder of the semester even though the colleges had obviated the need to stay in such housing. The universities themselves were quite grudgingly handing back dorm fees for the now non-existent dorm residents, but they relented after some clamor from students. In a word, continuing to pay rent and dorm costs was primary, the students' health was secondary. It should be clear that returning home to one's family, which is what students did, was safer in terms of the coronavirus than staying elsewhere with others in close quarters.

Landlords generally have been attempting to evict tenants who lost a job and cannot pay the rent. They have changed their locks and turned off utilities. New local edicts tried to prevent that during the pandemic.

As a consequence of stay-at-home, computer stores quickly depleted their stock. Even those who could afford good computers were hard put to find one soon to continue the work in their classes (and these students competed with a great number of parents who also sought more and better computers from stores in order to work from home, if they could work from home). That is referring to both college students and K-12 students.

Furthermore, all of a sudden a first grader's family had to decipher the new remote learning, since the first grader could not immediately do so. Teachers in K-12 were thrust as well into a new situation and the responsibility was put on them to somehow provide an education, and if not identical to what they were providing in the classroom before at least to provide a reasonable facsimile of it. Not only was that not the easiest thing to accomplish in a short time frame, now teachers faced another conundrum.

Namely the K-12 teachers discovered that remote learning and online education dictated greater allotments of their time to students, especially the younger ones who need a lot of assistance. So not only was there already inequality before the closing of schools, the inequality was exacerbated further given the new circumstances. Those circumstances involve the fact that some students are in a difficult situation at home without financial and other resources, which teachers now realized more starkly than they had before.

That this became so much the case was illustrated by the fact that many school districts simply decided to pass students from one grade to another due to the online problems. This type of passing is often otherwise known as social promotion. Social promotion is a term used by educators to designate the placement of students in the next grade who are not all that ready for it but hopefully mentally may adapt in a more positive way towards schooling. Retention in a grade generally leads to students losing hope and eventually dropping out in higher numbers as a result, which is not that positive for these students.

A new source of stress for the already stressed-out teachers pertained to the remote learning situations brought about by the pandemic. Specifically, they encountered frustrations in not being able to help sometimes those who needed help the most. Helping with homework just took on a whole different meaning. Before the virus there was much that students were given as work to do at home because there was not much time to convey new concepts, etc., during the regular class day. That should not have been the case, though teachers saw it as unavoidable. Homework was meant to be a review and reinforcement for what was taught in class. Understandably, many parents could not help their children with new concepts to be learned as homework, which is what homework had become the last several years.

Now, everything was homework: new concepts, review, and whatever teleconferencing that was possible under the circumstances. It is easy to see how teachers, students, and their parents were in newly stressful situations. Then, as if this were not a major problem, teachers and students were being called back to school in the fall of 2020 without clear protocols for the wearing of masks, social distancing, etc.

Teachers' unions representing the interests of the teachers had plenty to say about that. The tensions that teachers feel are about: the difficulty in teaching in a remote learning approach and environment (which is not ideal at all particularly for a good number of students) and then when school commences in the fall the possibility of their getting infected without precautions and guidance from administrators about safety and health issues.

Governor Abbott of Texas did not have anything of substance to say about the spike in infections after "opening" up the state, nor initially about teachers and their health and safety. The main thing he emphasized is that there was enough bed capacity in Texas for hospitalizations, as if to indicate that he is not as concerned about the pandemic as he is about opening up business and schools, since he states that the beds are there for those who consequently suffer. Then again, as soon as he said that, the beds weren't there. Houston essentially ran out of beds needed for COVID-19 patients. As if that was not enough to show his level of thinking, he also blamed young people for the infection rates, as if the young do what they do to cause problems for the rest of the state. This is his example of generational wars which are instigated every now and then when there is no basis for doing so, other than to distract from the economic failures of his and other like-minded cronies in society.

After all this he had to relent and decrease the activities of bars and restaurants in the summer during the spike in cases after having just opened them up for greater capacity. In other words, he had closed all nonessential businesses, then opened them up, then closed some again.

Trump said, moreover, what Abbott chose not to publicly or overtly say in the summer, that he (Trump) thought there should not be more testing for the virus because all this made the U.S. look bad (of all things). To be clear, the problem is not one of more testing, since the infection rate is higher than the testing rate. It is also very clear, though, that both of them and many others in political office are much more concerned with the optics of it all, the image of Texas and the U.S., particularly for "business climate" and economic purposes.

Nonetheless, the poorer high schoolers were already the ones more likely to be the ones dropping out before the pandemic, often to financially help support their family. The mitigation efforts which resulted in parents losing their jobs signify that helping to support the family takes on a new meaning as well. Moreover, tension from economic problems contributes to divorce (which is why it is higher among the poor). This also means that more single parents, even of toddlers, will have to work when there isn't much work available. Thus, their older sons and daughters might drop out of school to look for work.

Now teachers will be hard pressed to review more material at the start of school, from the previous grade, than they did before for the first couple of weeks as they usually did at the start of a new school year. They were already doing so particularly with poorer students who did not have the enrichment opportunities and resources such as those of some cognitively engaging activities and more extensive travel that better-off students have during the summer. The poorer youngsters thereby fall further behind by the end of summer. It may be October or later by the time the catching up occurs, at which time teachers will now have a shorter time span to teach the current grade level for the year, everything still falling behind what it should be.

Thus, it became clear that providing a K-12 education encountered unforeseen obstacles such as the above. However, not the least of these was that more work was asked of teachers and in fact was demanded of them, what with the expectation that these teachers be available almost around the clock in the online and remote learning mode to assist students, as some college students expect online professors to be at their beck and call at all hours.

In addition, teachers were calling students who did not have reliable internet services at home and of course were calling them for other reasons. They would talk not only with the students but also perhaps with the parents to see why schoolwork was not submitted, for example. That is a lot of calling, a lot of contacting people at various hours, a new normal of being almost a "round the clock" tutor to each student. Unsurprisingly, teachers were now more drained than they were before the virus. The new uncompensated speed up was also encountered in other occupations, of those who still had occupations.

It is not all that feasible for elementary school teachers to teach by phone 20 students adequately by calling every single one of them every school day. This is not to mention that this means the student or more likely the parent in the case of kindergarten and first graders will not be able to answer or talk with the teacher at a given time or be able to comprehend the assignments that easily by phone/online. It is difficult enough to communicate some lessons in the classroom. Now the situation is compounded for these professionals by having to do all this in an unwieldy way by phone and by computer.

An additional major problem is that poverty-stricken school districts already were heavily burdened with practically insurmountable problems, such as lack of materials which the better-off school districts have. There is also the lack of adequate nutrition for students to keep them attentive all day, to mention another problem or two.

In poor communities there are food deserts, as an example. This is where supermarkets stocked with nutritious, low cost food are scant, though there are plenty of convenience stores and McDonalds around.

Nonetheless in recognition of nutrition problems more school districts were starting to provide free school lunches and breakfasts to all students regardless of income, instead of being income eligible before that to qualify for the programs. Now that effort may become questionable with the lesser income of many who were without paid work during the lockdown, meaning less money for the schools to operate those programs from tax revenue.

Simply put, school districts derive in most cases almost half of their revenue from local taxes and property valuations. Much of the other half is from the state, and the remaining small amount is from the federal level, from federal taxes. In a word, the entities which are better off have more for their schools and those that are poorer have less, now substantially less with people being unemployed and not paying much in the way of taxes, either in federal income taxes or in the local and state sales taxes on items they buy.

The unemployed will not be able to buy much other than food (unless they go into heavier debt, which they cannot much do so anyway because of their declining credit ratings). Food is generally not taxed. Not much revenue results from this situation going into local and state coffers.

In fact, many agencies and institutions will be receiving less funding from local, state, and federal sources, while at the same time more money is needed to counteract the predicament of the coronavirus particularly in hospitals. Many hospitals were deriving much of their revenue from profitable elective and similar procedures/surgeries, with such profit now substantially lost for some time. Lo and behold, this became clear during the pandemic, while the public assumed that hospitals garnered their income/profit predominantly from treating sick people. Treating sick people is not as profitable as elective surgeries.

In K-12, the wealthier students are in the opposite situation than the situation the poorer ones face. The temporariness of online learning is easier to cope with for the wealthier, though it is not ideal as the classroom circumstances are for them. They and their parents harbor no anxiety about falling behind in school. White parents particularly have the resources of higher income, better education, and less discrimination against said parents.

Poorer ones and those of color do not enjoy these resources to weather them through it all. That is not to mention that students from wealthier families attend the better schools that have more resources as well and where teachers therefore do not encounter as many difficulties in contrast to teachers at poorer schools.

It was found that in K-12 and in college there were not uncommon instances of teachers and professors just transmitting in a clerical manner batches of assignments they found somewhere and were not necessarily creating assignments, etc. All of this was in order to quickly comply when pressured with the courses now having to be online. Teachers and professors did not get much guidance in a short matter of time from administrators. The support systems too often do not materialize when needed.

In continuing to mitigate the spread of the virus the inequalities will become more entrenched, since some variant of virtual/online/remote learning will be maintained to keep from too much contact among teachers and students. All this is at the expense of poorer whites and students of color who are in more troubling circumstances regarding that type of learning. It must be reiterated that in higher education poor students and those of color benefit more than even white students from courses in the classroom than from the second-rate online type.

Online courses have been offered for at least the past twenty years at the collegiate level, and still have not caught fire with students, with good reason. Most universities have nominal numbers of such courses, and even fewer degrees which are online, unless an institution of higher learning is exclusively online. However, there is much fraud in the latter, with thousands of students having their tuition recuperated and some online colleges going bankrupt and/or closing as a result of numerous problems.

Still, the teachers were not paid for that extra, stressful work and this unforeseen nonpayment for the extensive provision of services at all hours was not something they signed up for when they became educators. Some teachers struggled in trying to figure out why particular students were not doing the work through remote learning, and in the process realized that, for example, domestic violence was sometimes the case (calls to domestic violence centers increased with the stay-at-home directives). This was not that surprising, given the fact that parents and students were unexpectedly isolated and spent inordinate amounts of time together at home under stressful circumstances, particularly given the increase in unemployment. Joblessness results in the inability to pay bills, etc., leading to quarrels in families, to say the least.

Some of the child abuse may not be noticed now, as it was noticed by teachers when the children were in school. It is the emergency rooms that notice it now, often the more severe forms of abuse, such as broken bones, etc. There may not be many witnesses to the abuse at home. The future is uncertain about this and other related issues, particularly if schools again close for mitigation purposes.

Teachers' unions sought to address these new problems of teachers without much success. It should be noted that these educators already were doing much work that was unpaid. Now they were burdened with more, to include what seemed like nonstop, perhaps superfluous teleconferencing with administrators who micromanaged them, or simply had them attend more meetings if you will.

Regardless, the unionized teachers are not allowed to have a large, metal placard in front of the school as the military is. The military put these up stating they support that school, when it is nothing of the kind in comparison to teachers' unions, but their placard does function as a recruiting tool for students, parents, and teachers to see every single day. Even businesses get into the act and give out trinkets as tokens of support, of course to publicize their business. The failed Drug Awareness and Resistance Education, DARE, gives out rulers to students.

Already before the virus half of all who started teaching left teaching within five years, one third within three years. The probability may arise that those in teacher education in college may become more circumspect about getting that degree now. It is certainly not uncommon to experience burnout in the teaching profession with the myriad sources of stress and tension, which in turn they might bring back to their own families. In Finland and other countries teachers are respected along with physicians and are highly paid, with plenty of resources. They teach whatever they deem important to teach, since that is what technically a professional person should be doing, and they are accurately seen as professionals in that country.

Most teachers like teaching itself and are happy when they see progress in students, when there is progress. However, now they may wind up doing what some nurses are doing. Quite a number of nurses perceive that they are not provided with the support and equipment to do what they deem is necessary in a safe and healthy way without perhaps getting infected with the coronavirus and passing on the infection to their family, as has happened with a number of health care workers.

A health care worker, though, is now lauded as a hero. That hero designation can become vacuous when there is a very high risk of infection due to the misdeeds of administrators and others. Then infection can occur and is passed on to loved ones. So, some nurses quit. Many of these heroes were not provided adequate masks and other precautions against the virus, but were left to fend on their own and lauded with the appellation of heroes, in reality an empty gesture without material backup.

The reference to nurses, and others in health care, as heroes does not relieve the stresses they face. Recognition without compensation for the hazards is an empty gesture. The second thoughts about careers that those in the health profession such as nurses and physicians already had before the virus previously had led to these occupational gaps, filled by those from foreign countries. Basically, the pay, respect, and benefits of the health profession have not been up to par in too many instances.

This is without pointing out the financial situation of patients who cannot pay, while other countries provide health care without regard to the wallet or purse of the patient.   The health profession, including psychiatrists and others, know full well that the stress associated with the inability to afford needed health care breaks down the immune system, causing further deleterious effects on patients. All of this contributes to more and graver illness for those patients, and therefore more problems for everyone else. No one in society is completely isolated from the compounding of health problems.

It remains to be seen how many teachers therefore will come to see things the way some in the health profession increasingly do. Already significant numbers of teachers are retiring early because they are no longer able to work closely with students in the professional way they did before the virus. Additionally, older teachers would be more susceptible to infection.

It is uncertain how many of these retirees will be replaced with less experienced teachers, given the new problems from the pandemic of those who might enter the occupation. This is not to mention the new health risks from the virus for all teachers and staff at schools. With that being the situation, teachers who would want to leave teaching for another job may find it is not easy to find one in this economy of high unemployment and uncertainty regarding the health risks of other jobs.

The public supports teachers but a number of those in political office do not and in fact demonize teachers, especially since many teachers belong to teachers' unions. Unions are anathema to Trump and his followers. He does not have teachers very much in mind when emphasizing the re-opening of K-12. To put it another way he does not even have workers very much in mind in his references to re-opening the economy, but he does have in mind the business owners and corporations. Oblique references by him about workers really pertain to them as earners, that is, for corporate profit from consuming and as political pawns for Trump's re-election.

There are certain fields in education that the necessary closing of schools exacerbated. Special Education is one of those. Not only is it difficult to get and keep teachers in this field, these teachers now had greater problems in trying to educate in a remote manner these students. There are Special Ed students with severe problems that require sustained attention who were now at home with their (newly unemployed) parents and it became more difficult to tend to their special needs. Some of these students even require medication and definitely a lot of understanding and skills from teachers in this field. These students in a word require very close attention and holding sometimes, now made more difficult with the possibility of teachers getting infected by the students or vice versa.

In the elementary grades in particular teachers often hugged students and these hugs were the only ones some of the students got on a given day. A hug now has the greater possibility, though not necessarily probability, of dire consequences because of the virus. The hugs were so positive that a professor, Leo Buscaglia, left his position as a professor to give lectures and presentations to the public about hugging others and the endorphins and other neural transmitters released in so doing which are healthy.

The theory behind Buscaglia is sound but in practice it may be a problem now. Teachers and students hugging each other unfortunately may decline significantly. Undoubtedly there is a likelihood that policies will be developed about all this, lest a school district be sued for somehow causing a death via infection from hugging.

There are quite a number of situations that are now questionable in K-12. Contact sports such as football require frequent physical contact with each other. In band students sit close to each other. In choir there is the possible spewing infected droplets/aerosols. Parents who crowded together in auditoriums to see their youngster in a play now may not do as they did before, with the same applying to those going to see them perform in stadiums as well. Sons and daughters like to see parents and friends in an audience. Now with masks they are not quite recognizable in the auditorium.

Moreover, in stadiums many yell during the games, spouting more infectious droplets to others, with potentially serious consequences if they are not six feet away from each other and with masks. An odd picture would be fans sitting six feet apart yelling with masks on in stadiums.

In all these and other situations people cannot be six feet apart from each other all the time. It is questionable that coaches will refrain from close contact with their student athletes. Neither coaches nor players are going to wear masks where they cannot be heard in the field, nor are they going to wear gloves to any significant extent. Particularly in contact sports, masks and gloves would be a contradiction in terms. This is the case whether such sports would be at the K-12 level, collegiate, or pro.

A vaccine, treatment, and testing will not entirely resolve the possibility of infection. Testing for the virus, for example, cannot be administered for the entire school every day, including teachers, staff and students. It is not that feasible even once a week, since someone may get infected the next day after testing or during the interval of a week and thereby infect others during that time.

Simply put, teachers and students had been in constant contact with each other, and masks will not resolve much under these circumstances either. Some people cannot be heard when talking at a normal volume with a mask on, and teachers and students of course need to talk very much with each other to understand each other.

Some of this is pertinent to the college classroom also in that students and professors need to be distinctly heard, and talking with a mask can obviate this. In the college classroom there cannot be many classes with students six feet apart. Contact sports are common in universities also, as well as band, etc., with all the new attendant problems due to the virus. Discussions in the classroom at the collegiate level can be extensive with students interacting with each other either in class or outside class. Furthermore, not only do college students ask questions in class or comment, at times they approach the professor at close range with questions after class as well and in the office.

Since the idea is that both students and professors do much of their work on their own initiative and may interact with each other for only a few hours, that is different than the K-12 teachers who interact closely with their students for several hours every day. The norm for undergraduates is two hours of study for every hour of class time, while for graduates it is three hours for every hour of class time. In college interaction is less and for only the length of a course for three or so months though with more students in classrooms and lecture halls. K-12 teachers interact with their charges longer per day but with a smaller number of students, particularly at the elementary level. Still, this is for a long nine months of the school year with the same students even when switching a class or two. Thus, the infection possibilities vary for higher education and K-12.

This means that teachers will now have greater anxiety because of their generally intense levels of interaction. This would affect anyone's teaching ability, particularly in schools in areas with a higher incidence of infection and thus higher anxiety. The teaching/learning may suffer. The outcome is similar to the teaching/learning that suffers in areas with higher rates of poverty, all these constraints affecting the evaluation/promotion of teachers and therefore their morale.

The worry for professors, on the other hand, is the much greater numbers of students they have than K-12 classes do throughout the academic year and therefore the greater possibility to interact with the larger numbers, emphasizing here the "possibility" since too many college students do not interact much with their professors anyway. They may become less interested in interacting with professors and others now, given social distancing. Close interaction and collaboration with professors may decline.

College students come and go more easily in the higher education setting, literally, than in K-12. That is, not only do they sometimes leave in the middle of a semester (or even in the middle of a lecture) and drop a class or classes, they may not return in a particular semester, or drop out of college and re-enroll years later or never again. Additionally, there are so many activities in the larger colleges that students there interact with many different people, in dining halls, dorms, activities they attend (including extracurricular ones) and so forth. It would be almost impossible to determine a carrier who is transmitting the virus. Too many encounters in higher education are of a fleeting kind, even if within six feet of each other prior to the coronavirus.

The higher education circumstances are not at all that common in K-12. In the latter case laws indicate they need enroll in school at least through age 16, and are even considered truant if they do not have a legitimate excuse for an absence. Clearly that does not apply to higher education, though professors can require attendance for a grade. Many do not require that.

In some courses, college students introduce themselves on the first day of class and usually say where they are from, but some now might hesitate on this. Those from New York City might fear being shunned. College students here from Italy or Spain might sense others grimacing if they say they are from those countries. The same applies to students from China. Woe to the student who says he or she is from Wuhan. There still are white college students who switch their seating away from blacks. Now some might move away from those hailing from the above and other hometowns. Instead of college being a welcoming environment, that may change somewhat.

The areas of study might change in comparison to the previous situations. Specifically, those who had an interest in being a nurse, an EMT, a school teacher, a police officer, a physical therapist and other areas of interest in higher education where they work very closely with others might have second thoughts about those certifications and degrees. As often happens with cycles of interests, if there were to be fewer students interested in such areas, there would develop a dearth in those majors and occupations. Then there would be a greater need for those types of students and perhaps more would thereafter enroll in those areas. That had been the case with some fields before the virus. Now some majors may see a permanent dearth.

Whether some careers might be considered which include a coronavirus occupational hazard is another matter, but that is currently the great need at this time. Some teachers have been asking (and receiving sometimes) for what in the military is called combat pay because of some very difficult or even hazardous/dangerous situations they face every day, in contrast to other teachers.

There are more immediate concerns now in education. Though there appears to be a necessity in mitigation efforts for professors, teachers, and students to wear masks and gloves, this is an unlikely scenario in the sense that not everyone will do so all the time while in school/college. The question arises whether even principals and superintendents will do so. From the top of society, Trump never much did though he had others around him wearing masks. Directives work when practiced, not when they are on paper only without teeth, without a fine and other consequences for flouting them.

Chapter 4

Religion

Because of directives to stay at home, church attendance was an anomaly for many weeks for most people, but not all. A social change consequential to this is that church members may come to realize more than they did before that they do not need a church building to worship on Sunday or any day. That this was for camaraderie or other reasons more so than for worship, praying, and reading the Bible is now perhaps realized. Perhaps still not. For a good number of churchgoers, any Christian message is lost five minutes after the service on the way home anyway, a swift retrogression into non-Christianity.

All of this is in addition to the decline of mainline churches. Many in the congregation were less than fervent already, and now may shed their official membership altogether. They will question, additionally, why they should attend church and possibly get infected and thereby infect a family member as well, who may die.

The same logic is evinced in regard to other institutionalized settings, such as sports games in stadiums, etc. If such fans attend they may likewise get infected, even if there is a vaccine available and treatment. Being elbow to elbow is may not necessarily that significant an aspect of church service anymore, nor perhaps of attending sports games, etc. Singing at church is practically banned, since doing so expels more droplets with the louder voices.

On the other hand there is the rapid rise of those who classify themselves as having no religious preference, which is now the largest category in religious classification in the U.S. (larger than any other specific category of religion). No religious preference is not about being irreligious, though, since many of this segment of the population have some religious beliefs, but rather that they do not prefer to formally belong to any one church. Then there are those who are atheist or agnostic. In a word, religion itself is being more swiftly transformed today because of the virus than was the case before.

There was also another category of those who when they did attend did so at a non-denominational place of worship. Of course, there was a large segment of Christians who engaged in televangelism (electronic religion, per the sociological nomenclature) and consequently did not attend a church at all. Televangelism is often non-denominational in order to attract as many as possible, with an emphasis on donations to stay on the air. Yet even televangelists have a congregation present for the cameras, which now may be awkward without many of the said followers panned by cameras in their seats due to the virus. Empty seats do not make for very good optics.

All this may not bode well for official, organized mainline churches, or other places of worship to begin with, when it is realized that Christianity can be practiced from home, as many other things such as jobs and school were in 2020. Just as there are going to be more jobs where employees work from home now and more online, remote learning types of education, there will be more worship not just from home but from anywhere. Many churches now provide online church services and advertise that. Of course, it was that or nothing in the interim to maintain a semblance of church worship.

As a consequence of these matters, the lack of Christianity among a number of pastors is laid bare now. The number one tenet of Christianity is doing for others. Yet some pastors have not energetically told their congregations to stay home from church, which is after all in the best interest of the congregants' health. Some ministers apparently had a greater concern not for them but for the decline in contributions to the church and the optics of it all without a congregation present, as if people could not pray in their home for the time being.

As has been very often said before by many other writers (including Christian writers), many churches themselves would not welcome Christ among them, what with Christ saying that it is more likely that a camel would pass through the eye of a needle than a rich person go to heaven, and numerous other such statements throughout the Bible.

Perhaps when members of some congregations see what their pastor did at the beginning of the virus crisis they may not be interested in church attendance much anymore, unless they go along with the pastors' hypocrisy.

Then again, some pastors admonish their congregation that they need not worry about a virus, that if their faith is strong enough they will not be infected. Likewise these pastors are not unlike the snake ("serpent") handling sects who believe that their faith will keep them from being bitten. Yet, some of them have indeed been bitten and even died. However, those who die are relegated to those whose faith was not strong enough.

Today some of those who believed they would not get infected if their faith was strong enough did get infected, analogous to the script of the snake handlers. This is not germane only to Christians. Those of any given faith believe they are the true faith, as do those who are Buddhist, Islamic, Jewish, Hindu, etc., alongside the countless sects within each of these, and others. These various believers perceive the coronavirus in their own light.

It will be interesting to see how many of the congregants will be six feet apart throughout the service when attending, with masks and gloves. Not many were when churches re-opened. There is not room in some churches for the members to be six feet apart from each other unless the services are greatly multiplied and sequential. Most important, congregations may come to see that love for each other is more paramount than having to stand shoulder to shoulder with strangers in church and perhaps get infected in the process and die. There is a point during the Catholic mass when parishioners shake hands with all of those around them. If that was considered as necessary before, it may not be so anymore. Things change. It was a sin to eat meat on Fridays for Catholics a few decades ago, then it was not a sin. There is a problem when something is said to be a sin and then that it is not a sin, and this from the main Christian group in the U.S.

Some businesses (profit-making ventures) such as Hobby Lobby which considered itself very Christian kept its doors open while other businesses closed. That said something about them at the time and they were trying to prove some kind of point. They wound up shuttering after all along with everyone else.

The pastors who proclaim to conquer the virus have not only not done so, some members of their congregation may very well die from infection. A miracle from any pastor, any minister, has yet to materialize along these lines for their congregation and be documented. When and if the virus subsides to an extent, and/or a vaccine and a treatment come about they will state that it was because of their beseeching. This is tantamount to much of what Trump does, taking credit for whatever is perceived as positive that occurs, in order to appear triumphant.

As in the case of the flu, vaccines are not necessarily a complete success and there is no definitive cure for the flu for everyone and never has been. The likelihood is that the spread of the coronavirus will be mitigated, but not eliminated, with deaths still occurring. The cliché, which Trump has repeated in a flippant, obligatory manner, is that one death is one too many. Obviously there have been and will continue to be many more than one death. Evidently empathy is not his forte (nor that of stone-faced Pence), using Christianity as a prop when expedient when he pictured himself in front of a church with a Bible in hand. Trump and Pence give religion a bad name. The one saving grace of both of them is that they make it possible for society to demarcate quite glaringly now the two camps basically in society: those seeking to maintain the socioeconomic power they have (and as proxies for the president), and the rest of society.

Nonetheless, the societal changes due to the virus will persist even if there had been a few thousands of deaths. It goes without saying that this is not even discussing the social changes in the poorer countries and their situation now or in the future. Their future is significantly intertwined with ours in a number of ways. The poor in the third world grasp at straws from the first world. All countries are interdependent, though some to a greater or lesser extent. What is impractical is isolationism.

Religions' idealism is a focus on others. However, some of the religious will perhaps come to believe that (after a keeping of distance from each other) they do not need others all that much. Less concern for others may predominate, all this morphing into more loneliness.

Loneliness is a subjective feeling, whereas being alone is an objective circumstance whereby a person is not in the company of others. Not all that many will now be too enthusiastic about helping those who are sick. Christ commanded his followers to tend to the sick and the downtrodden. The proverbial going to a neighbor for a cup of sugar is disappearing with the appearance of the coronavirus. Even the elderly who identified themselves as Christian were not voting much for school bonds, under the assumption that, well, these kids are not their kids.

The kids of many white elderly are all grown up. Said elderly white are dying off in comparison to the increase of those younger who are of color. In part because of this, generational "wars" are instigated by those in political office and by some in the media. In sum there is not much Christian regard for all. The false "wars" divert attention from overall inequality and related problems.

It is, though, a matter of class conflict in society when there is funding for the wealthy (including corporate welfare) as well as funding for war profiteers and the military-industrial complex that President Eisenhower himself warned us against right before he left office. As Senator Durbin has emphasized, bankers run Congress. That was a stark public admission, though otherwise it has been known for a long time. Woodrow Wilson had said the same some 100 years ago. The latter added that the much larger class of workers were needed to do the manual work in society for the smaller number (presumably the wealthy).

Thus the lack of concern for others, in this case for their health, is seen in the fact that some Christian church members opted to host religious home services, prayers, and the like, with the emphasis here on groups in these homes in defiance of social distancing. Thus, it is questionable that some consider themselves so Christian that the first rule of doing for the betterment of others is ignored, in this case pitting the health concerns of other people against what some members want. This is too often synonymous with what Trump wants, such as when he was striving to see the churches full on Easter Sunday, no matter the death toll from that. All this speaks volumes about many so-called Christians.

Either we do the positive, such as dealing constructively with the virus and many benefit, or we do the negative and many suffer. It is not complicated. Since the U.S. refers itself in name as largely Christian even though many recent presidents do not even go to church, the country does not follow the basic Christian precepts of doing for others.

When some things are done, after all, it is too often for profiteering purposes. Instead of being concerned in a Christian sense of doing for the meat packers, some in political office ordered them back to work after closure of the plants for mitigation purposes. Returning them back was for the profiteering of meat packing companies.

Farmworkers are not even an afterthought for Christians. When farmworkers pack fruit and vegetables in produce companies they work shoulder to shoulder akin to meat packers on a daily basis. Many of the farmworkers are undocumented and are the lowest of the lowly in society. That says a lot about a lack of Christianity in society.

Chapter 5

Sports

Already in the spring of 2020 there was much fear and loathing among college sports people and the prospects for the upcoming fall. Much the same applies to collegiate football as it does to pro football, with a major exception. Football in college in many ways brings more revenue to colleges than any other of their sports. The anxieties became palpable when cutbacks in pay for football athletic staff were announced in the spring. That assumes there will be some semblance of football in the fall, what with "social distancing," masking (?) of fans in the stadium, of players on the field (?), etc.

Trump himself brought up the NFL in the spring of 2020 in the middle of the skyrocketing deaths from the pandemic. This indicated his anxiety which in turn reflected the anxiety of the NFL itself regarding an existential threat to the profits of the NFL and the very meaning of pro football, what with its association with the military and all things patriotic, among other things (of course Trump even mentioned the role of the military in the pandemic much more so than he mentioned the civilian health care workers).

Basically, huge profits of the NFL are at stake, and these profits could plummet with less attendance at games and less buying of pro football paraphernalia (from less interest in the games and the teams). There already was a decline in attendance at football games, both pro football and college, in the seasons prior to the pandemic.

It will be interesting to see how much scoffing occurs among rabid fans about changes in football game protocols. Specifically, it would be interesting to have TV spectators see stadiums as a sea full of masked fans seating six feet apart with gloves on, or on the contrary the stadium with fans elbow to elbow, yelling and thus spewing out possibly contagious aerosols and droplets, without masks and gloves. The former is not good for NFL imagery and profits, while the latter is OK for the profiteering of NFL owners (with infections and deaths rising, that is).

It would seem to be incongruous to bring up the NFL in April by Trump and others all that much in relation to the virus, without indicating much else about the league (such as the spring draft of players) in the middle of April of 2020. However, the reality of monumental failures in the NFL season in the fall of 2020 signify much more than meets the eye, which is why there is so much anxiety.

What was discussed above pertaining to forms of regional discrimination, and thus differential treatment, has been the case in the sports world, particularly in pro football as well. Specifically, as a poignant example, the Dallas Cowboys and their rabid fans have had nothing but disdain historically against northerners. The origin of this is the defeated Confederate states. The South then had to tolerate the northerners they referred as carpetbaggers, because they supposedly put their belongings in a carpet they rolled up to come South during Reconstruction. Some of these northerners were teachers who taught black students, and some of these teachers and others were murdered by southerners. Those southerners who helped the carpetbaggers were referred to as scalawags, pejoratively so even in Texas schoolbooks. Today whites who help blacks are often referred to in a pejorative way as well, as race traitors.

For many years the chief rivals of the Cowboys thus were the Redskins (wouldn't you know it they are from Washington DC), with their name changing soon. Another rival for the rabid fans of the Cowboys are the New York Giants, since New Yorkers as also mentioned above have been disdained to an extent before in the South, but currently even more so in a form of discrimination against them due to the higher numbers of virus cases in comparison to other places in the country recently.

Now that those two teams are not that much of competitive rivals (actually losers lately) in the Eastern Division (which includes Dallas, which is obviously in the southern U.S., not the East) in pro football being weak overall, well another rival has risen to take their place lately, the Philadelphia Eagles, now earning the Cowboys fans' ire not only for being in the disdained northern environs but particularly now that the Eagles have sort of a winning team.

Much of this pertains to demographics. Texas is the second most populous state after California, and is the largest in area and the most populous in the ever-meaningful South. The state has four of the top eleven most populous cities in the U.S. The majority population of the state is comprised of people of color, while about three quarters of the school population is as well (children are the future of the state, whereas whites in all demographic categories are declining).

Texas is also the state where some of the most crucial social issues in the U.S. have eventuated, such as those of affirmative action, bilingualism, the undocumented, and voter ID, among others. There is a high level of anxiety that whites harbor about all this in the state, not the least of reasons being that whites are fast declining in population while people of color are increasing in population.

Additionally, the Cowboys are in Dallas, the city with one of the highest rates of inequality in the country, which belies the shiny media image. It has consistently been considered the most dangerous or one of the most dangerous cities in Texas, which itself has a violent past in every respect of its history. It is income inequality which is the major predictor of homicides, and the city has high rates of both, inequality and homicides and as such is one of the most bloodthirsty in the nation.

In a word the city remains among the top ten in the in the nation in types of inequality in all major facets of society. The police, for one, have been a perennial problem for blacks. An attempt to ameliorate that was made when Texas state highway patrol troopers were brought in to the city. They worsened the racism against blacks. Troopers likewise have against Latinos historically throughout the state, particularly by the Texas Rangers, who are an arm of the state troopers. The Dallas Cowboys games essentially are a handy coverup for problems which Dallas and the state have, and the team serves that purpose admirably.

Somehow there is an understanding that with so many of the players being black, this is just fine with the Cowboys in Texas, so to speak, as if to indicate that the city and the state are a beacon for racial equality because of the team members. This bears a similarity with Tony

Romo as a Latino who did not make it a habit of emphasizing that he was Latino, yet Latinos gleefully rooted for him in large part because of his background.

Similarly in a political sense many Latinos voted for Ted Cruz, since he is Latino, though they were not clear that he is Cuban. The tiny percentage (3) among Latinos of Cuban Americans in the nation, or the state for that matter, have never been interested in the much larger group of Latinos in the nation, those of Mexican origin (65%). Thus, the latter were fooled by Cruz. Immigration by Cubans is political, yet that of Mexicans immigrating here is economic.

Then along comes Abbott the current governor. In campaigning he flaunted to Latinos his Latina wife, as well as conveying to voters that he is in a wheelchair. Both factors have been shown to be meaningless in terms of Abbott's policies and efforts as governor of that state. But it all helped in getting elected, and again many were fooled, particularly Latinos.

Abbott's policies regarding the coronavirus are virtually identical to white Trump's in his anxieties more so about the lack of profiteering in the state than about the health of Texans. Abbott was absolutely forced to go from masking in the state, to not masking, then again to masking recently. The mirage of progress under Abbott for voters evaporated soon after election, as if this had not been a tale foretold. This is the Texas of the Cowboys, and Abbott and others are delighted for the opiate service from the Cowboys for the people of Texas.

Parenthetically it should be added that being a person of color and/or a woman does not inherently mean that these will do anything in particular for the downtrodden. In addition to Cruz being an example of that, there are women such as Hillary Clinton and Madeleine Albright as examples in regard to women. The former referred to young blacks as super predators and was brutal with them in her husband's criminal justice reform, while the latter was all right with hundreds of thousands of Iraqi children dead as a result of U.S. sanctions.

Very importantly, likewise with the coronavirus there is a greater likelihood that, say, a black official would be more concerned about the impact of the virus on blacks, if only because a black official may have some similar experiences as other blacks. As an example, those of color and women did not support the Iraq war to the level that white men did. Still, there is no guarantee, nothing inherent, however, of that genuine concern for blacks by a black, ditto of a woman for women, etc. That must be kept in mind about anyone speaking about the coronavirus or other matters.

(It needs to be added, though, in a different way, that often immigrants of color may not see or want to see the racism here, perhaps because things were different in their country of origin. Nevertheless, in a few years they come around to realizing the racism here.)

Now the aforementioned New York team will moreover be taunted, though maybe not too overtly to avoid appearing callous, by the Cowboys fans for the initially high coronavirus rates in that state. So, disdain will now be added to discrimination directed against New Yorkers, whether by Cowboys fans and/or society in general. Already the negative perceptions were harbored by those in the South in general against New Yorkers.

Even though the Cowboys have not even gone to the Super Bowl in over twenty years (though every year their mantra of entitlement is claimed: "Next year the Super Bowl!"), yet the media is desperate in maintaining the moniker for them of America's Team for no good reason. It just seemed some thirty years ago or so that some of their fans supposedly were seen in various parts of the country at the time, which can be said of any team, yet there was no quantification of it in any way.

That's it, a sports media creation if ever there was one, to salve the nerves of those in the state that has some of the most severe social problems, an opiate for the people of Texas. Of course, the lives of the fans are sort of left in limbo in the off season, being as how life is breathed back into them every August. Alongside this, for those dubious of the opiate effect, WWE, World Wrestling Entertainment, was designated an essential service in Florida to sooth nerves (and it was explicitly claimed as doing that for the fans) when other entities remained in lockdown mode.

This was similarly the case in Roman times, though with people thrown to the lions for entertainment (distraction) purposes for the spectators and their problems. Even Dr. Anthony Fauci, of all people, felt he had to mention the circumstances of the NFL in relation to the coronavirus. That is how desperate he, Trump, and others are to sometimes distract from the pandemic, not to mention that the NFL per se throughout the country distracts from and covers up societal problems such as poverty and racism.

Quite significant is that the team's players presumably represent something about Dallas, or about Texas, or whatnot. To the contrary, they do not represent anything about Texas (there are the Houston Texans team, but instead the Cowboy imagery is everywhere in the state), and the Cowboys could care less. They are team members, as all other players elsewhere are, for the money they get ("pro," professional football players, only in terms of playing for big money, since a professional in the technical sense of the word is completely otherwise).

Technically, a professional person is one who has a graduate degree, years of experience, and one whose judgment is independent, and in that manner utilizes his expertise and is respected for it, whether paid highly or not. The term really does not apply to someone who engages in some activity (football, gambling, etc.) for big money. The definition of professional has been changed by the public as has the sociological definition of social distance.

Although Kaepernick was anathema to the owner of the Cowboys, Jerry Jones, the former won and has been vindicated in his kneeling for justice for blacks. He did so to indicate that the third stanza of the anthem was in reference to blacks not having a refuge from slavery except for the gloom of the grave. Likewise, Muhammad Ali was ultimately vindicated when the Vietnamese defeated the U.S. The Army drafted him and he refused the induction, saying that no Vietnamese had used a racial slur against him and that blacks here had more in common with the Vietnamese people than with American warmongers.

It is clear that blacks have made a connection among the following: their higher death rates from the pandemic, their higher unemployment rate after closings in the economy due to the pandemic, coincident with their higher death rates/brutality at the hands of police. All this is related to the issues Kaepernick, Ali, and many others have brought up.

In sum, there is now a reality setting in, that those in power have lied to us. Finally, blacks and others have now seen how society had made fools of them for hundreds of years in the U.S. (and of others throughout the world as well), starting with the fraud of Columbus in regard to Native Americans.

One of these examples, the University of Texas song at football games, "The Eyes of Texas" has racist styes in those eyes. It originated from a minstrel show which in turn was associated with Confederate General Robert E. Lee. It is well known by some at UT that a president of UT, Prather, would tell others that the eyes of the South were glaring down on them.

It is interesting that other teams have also looked at the origins of their songs. They have seen the racist skeletons in the closets of owners, etc., as well. This constitutes a continuing education for American society about its true history, a history of inequality and about its former and current leaders, including the Founding Fathers as they are called and many others.

Whether there is much kneeling at games, pro football or otherwise, Jones and Trump will be even more nervous now about the optics of any players kneeling, particularly when the Commissioner of the NFL, Goodell, now supports the players who protest police brutality. It is interesting how this is playing out with the players, the great majority of them black, and to see Jones' reaction.

What is clear is that Jerry Jones has not said much at all about the protests lately, as most of the significant pro football people have. He failed in his opposition to Kaepernik. His concern is that he at least wants to uphold his squeaky clean image for the rabid fans of the Cowboys as America's Team for advertisers, the games, and buyers of the team's paraphernalia. It is a monetary concern. His vehement denunciation of Kaepernik was completely and purposely in line with Trump at the time. But the less rabid the fans may be now, the less the profit. He, the players, and fans are trying hard to blithely go on and not allow anything of significance to hinder them. Now they have the extra task, other than distracting from and covering up serious social problems, of soothing the nerves of unemployed fans who silently fear the coronavirus contagion.

Jones, like Trump, initially had not publicly shown any consternation about the coronavirus. Doing so (again as in the case of Trump) would mean having to address the serious consequences, only here it would be how it could possibly affect the pro football season. Apparently, the health of the players is not primarily a worry for the bottom line of pro football, other than to keep them healthy for that bottom line, sometimes even playing them while injured when a dose of pain killer keeps them mechanically going to the end of the game. Players can be replaced with others waiting in the wings. The players nurse serious lifelong injuries after their contracts expire, nonetheless.

Jones was adamant against any substantive discussion of concussion injuries to players. Doing so would sully the image of his team as well as pro football in general. Still, parents became increasingly less interested in football for their kids due to possible concussions. If the pipeline to pro football diminishes, along recently with the declining number of attendees even before the pandemic, that can spell catastrophe for pro football specifically and football as a violent sport in general. Jones seeks to maintain a pristine image of his team and the game when there is none.

Concussions also occur not only in football but also to a significant extent in the military, often serious injuries referred to as Traumatic Brain Injuries, TBI. When quite a number of soldiers suffered some of these injuries from a blast at a base, Trump minimized this by saying they just had developed some headaches from it.

Jones had mentioned that the head of Papa Johns Pizza was a person that he lauded. Jones did commercials for the pizza. That franchise had connections with the Cowboys throughout the Dallas-Fort Worth area. That pizza person is the same one who was said to have used a racial slur.

Thus, in addition to the fiascos that transpired because of the coronavirus in regard to pro football games, there is now the added reminder of the anthem and thereby the history of brutality against blacks to dampen pro football profits even further. There are various reminders to the owners that they have numerous blacks as players, without their respecting these blacks except as investments for profiteering. Of course, it cannot all appear to be too crass, so charity events are staged by team members, no different than the "coffee with a cop" and Blue Santa public relations stunts of police in communities, momentarily erasing thoughts of brutality, until the next case of brutality erupts in a video recording, that is.

With their normalization of their chauvinism it would be no surprise that owners and rabid fans would ridicule, along with the "open the state" propagators, much about the virus. The "open the state" protestors per se were overwhelmingly white, male, and Trump supporters sporting unabashedly his re-election signs, and some of them were waving the Confederate flag. (The Confederate flag, statues, bases named after Confederate leaders such as Ft. Hood in Texas, after the police brutality protests are being eliminated, as a top general and as Colin Powell said, and toppled because of the racism they symbolize).

Of interest, the "open the state" protestors at the time did not emphasize opening social agencies, schools, etc. Trump articulated for the protestors the opening of businesses, for profit for the employers and not for benefitting the public as public agencies would. These agencies, be they state, county or local also employed people who needed to go back to work. Many who work in these agencies, though, are unionized and Trump opposes unionized workers. Moreover, such agencies are non-profit, and again Trump is not interested in that, nor are others in political office.

To add to Trump's lack of concern for such employees, many who work in agencies and non-profits are black and Latino. It should go without saying that he does not have their interest at heart, as he evinced throughout his racist rants in his failed Tulsa rally and where social distancing and masks were a joke to the attendees and to him. He saw the attendees only as voters for him, as his base.

As if that were not enough to emphasize, many who work in agencies and non-profits are women. So, there is no great clamor for Trump's "open the state" proxies for these types of employees going back to work and to open up those types of places. He only demanded that schools open in the fall, without any mention of the unionized teachers as employees going back to work, though.

That speaks volumes about the chauvinism of the "open the state" protestors, as against others who are people of color and poor whites siding more so with mitigation efforts by the state. It was developing into a referendum on Trump whether to show support for him publicly by not wearing a mask, or oppose him by wearing one. Of course, the situation got out of hand when some Republican governors opened the state prematurely at the urging of the president, infections spiked, then these governors recommended that masks be worn, and finally capitulated and mandated that masks be worn in public places of business when the rate of infection got out of hand due to their failed policies.

Obviously, some people felt a burst of relief from cabin fever. Some at beaches were fined for not practicing social distance, but the "open the state" protestors were not touched by the police for failing to practice social distance (said protestors, again, were proxies for what Trump and the corporations sought). This is par for how the police approach whites versus those of color in protests. Thus, those who later on protested police brutality in part took their cue from what the police failed to do against the overwhelmingly white, and some armed, aforesaid protestors.

Anathema to rabid fans therefore would be to go to games, if they were allowed to attend, with mask, gloves, and be six feet apart. It remains to be seen how all this plays out, because even with a vaccine, treatment, testing, etc., and thus supposedly no more masks, gloves, and social distancing, there would still be the outside possibility of getting infected and thereafter infecting family members, with still an outside possibility of death, but nonetheless a possibility. It remains to be seen the level of risk some people will take. The virus will still be around, certainly in other parts of the world as well and the deaths from it, since vaccines, treatment, and testing will be unequally administered here and throughout the world.

Actually, in the spring of 2020 there were already efforts to eliminate the pro baseball season altogether. The reason is simple. The owners realized they were not going to get much profit otherwise, even from a shortened season, though some of them were still striving to put fans in the baseball park and sell the beer and merchandise. This is not all that different than when cattle owners slaughter cattle, dairy farmers pour milk down the drain, and wheat farmers burn their wheat if they all cannot get the price they want for their commodities, regardless of hunger. Given the confusion ensuing from the pandemic, then again some pro baseball owners sought to have some sort of shortened season, still up in the air and to be determined in the summer. The largely unspoken image of baseball as sort of representative of something about the U.S. versus the profits or lack thereof were the issues that snarled the pro baseball owners and many others in the country.

In a similar manner, the Olympics are not a representation of sportsmanship in the U.S. The same applies to other countries. It is basically an enterprise, an exercise in commercialization, from the competition to host the games to the advertising, etc. Other than the monetary focus, there is the chauvinism, such that each country and particularly the U.S. feels that they should be the winners in a sport, and that in winning it says something good about the people of the country. In fact, the media so focuses on the U.S. that in former days when the communist countries would win more medals than the U.S., the media would not emphasize that, but would when the U.S. won more medals. The chauvinistic and the commercial aspects of the Olympics are paramount, not sportsmanship. The latter is not even commented on by the sportscasters.

While the owners of pro sports were panicking to put fans in stadiums, etc., some pro players were opting out of playing. The players who are doing so in a variety of sports venues are those who are concerned about contracting the virus and infecting their families, such as a pregnant wife. There are other reasons, but very importantly those who opt to instead play are too often doing so because they need the money, not out of devotion to the team. There are some, such as basketball and baseball players, who increase their possibility of infection by playing a number of times a week in physical contact with other teams whereas in football it is once a week.

The optics of all this in pro sports, given the violence of football in particular, will be interesting. Moreover, the violence of pro football is of the same cloth as the military, who strut their own selves during the football games. It should be no surprise that media and political leaders glorified the military for their "help" in regard to the pandemic, not the least of reasons that this is good press for the military, better than a recruitment poster.

Somewhere in all this is the football widow, which refers to the woman who is basically ignored, a nonentity, for the duration of the football season. With the coronavirus and emphasis on staying at home, such widowhood will be exacerbated, with the relief only of the wife going somewhere outside the house with the prospect of catching the virus out there. Spousal expectations are that they are to pay some attention to each other, but this is too often nullified during football season. Not only on weekends would such expectations in a loving relationship be the case, now with college football on Saturdays and the NFL not only on Sundays but now on Mondays, Thursdays, etc., there is no relief in sight for the football widow.

As if these consternations were not enough, there were efforts before the virus to extend the NFL season, from the August preseason onward, of all things. Widowhood would be extended onto most of the year. In addition, a longer season leads to more injuries for the players, but they will just be spit out by the owner after that, useless and replaced immediately with a new one to be injured. All of this is not a very positive development for marriages and the spouses as players who facilitate the profiteering, etc. This costs some and benefits others.

Many see Super Bowl Sunday as a dangerous time for women. However, when women go to pro football games they usually go to accompany their men. Obviously, there are some women who know more about football than men and are more diehard fans than some men, but clearly it is the way around by a long shot.

There is a new dimension to the football season, though, since not only was attendance at football games already declining, the team owners will strive to not show the even emptier stadiums from here on in. More fans will be watching the game at home, there will be more football widows, and likely therefore more domestic violence from rabid fans seeing their teams lose, with members of the family nearby as handy targets for venting their frustrations.

By the way, not many of the remaining number of fans who attended the games will be able to do so now, for the simple reason that their economic situation will not allow it. This will decimate attendance even further. Obviously, their lesser or no income is likely a result of losing jobs during the closing of the economy in the spring of 2020, with many employers not calling them back, or calling them back at lower pay. It is easy for bosses to offer lower pay to desperate persons, and the latter will take such pay. The alternative is nothing in income for the foreseeable future, with unpaid bills facing them.

Naysayers of the economics/business of it all are in short order confronted with the very names of the stadiums (ATT for the Cowboys) and baseball fields (Minute Maid for the Astros) and the Nike swoosh and the like on players and others. The pervasive commodification indicates that countless ubiquitous symbols proclaim that everything is for sale, now more than ever. One can peruse a school yearbook from the 1950s clothing, etc., and not find such.

Football players and others have become sandwich board men, the term for those who in former times walked up and down a street advertising a business. One side of the board said something in front and the other said something else in back, both hanging on the individual hired to do that for the day.

With the precariousness of jobs now, the basis of consumerism will be reconsidered as never before. In essence, there are better things to do than getting unnecessary stuff is what the conclusion will be, further eroding and collapsing the economic ethos and system.

One of the other economic/consumer aspects of football is the football pot. This is another thing many look forward to in betting in a variety of ways on the game. In fact, in the Super Bowl there is even a bet that gamblers place on the outcome of the toss of the coin. In all this betting, the other facets of football, such as the violence, the football widow, and the consumerism of merchandise are part and parcel of the game. Betting is not an isolated activity, with these other facets somewhere alongside it.

The violent aspects of pro football and of the military per se contrasts sharply with what health workers, teachers, and others emphasize, which is life. That health workers, for example, are seen as heroes in signs displayed throughout the country is something that should have always been the case. Still, the media uses them as props in the media's individualization of such heroes, without further discussion about the macro aspects of health care. To put it another way we don't have affordable or free health care for everyone in the U.S., unlike elsewhere. For the media that point is a nonstarter for discussion, hence the individualization of the "heroes," squelching discussion of the macro, the large-scale issues of health care.

That the violence inherent in the military and in pro football is the case is evident in that the two are associated very closely. The media compromised itself, for example, during the invasion by the U.S. of Iraq with their use of imbedded journalists with the soldiers. Journalists were loath therefore to displease soldiers by showing bloodied and dying Americans, or by critique of the war for that matter. In pro football, the violence in the form of groans and screams is purposefully muted or deleted on national TV, unless it is a documentary on violence in football.

Journalists are similarly beholden to "America's Team" and generally would prefer not to displease that team which the media themselves a long time ago so christened. The media lauding the Cowboys is synonymous with a crowd somewhere chanting "USA! USA! USA!" to squelch and drown out detractors, be it protestors or whoever else is questioning anything.

Essentially therefore, the military (signifying death and violence) flyovers in games and the national anthem (signifying death for slaves) are part and parcel of pro football. During the games, military references are made to the blitz, the bomb, aerial assaults, etc. The source of the angst in Jerry Jones as the owner of the Cowboys is not difficult to discern once this is realized and when someone such as Kaepernick tinkers with any optics of the pro football of Jones and other owners.

Jones had shown that angst openly against Kaepernick before, but now may be keeping much of it to himself, lest he overturn the apple cart of his team and the league. The only other times he displays anxiety is when his team loses a bid in the playoffs to the Super Bowl, though he may not have realized he was being filmed at the time. The coronavirus has impacted pro football and the related Black Lives Matter protests: blacks are prominent in the games as well as in being brutalized by police and having very high unemployment rates due to losing jobs because of the virus. All this has modified some of the equations in the minds of team owners. Reevaluation is the order of the day.

Despite all this, the media trots out their "human interest" individualization. This is the same script employed in reference to societal problems, whether it is in regard to crime, terrorism, etc. An individual hero is found and lauded in such instances who supposedly saved lives in some way, without any reference to why there is crime, terrorism, etc., in the first place. The journalistic maxim of "if it bleeds, it leads" is primary, for profits but not enlightenment.

Chapter 6

The Economy

Less taxes collected due to the Depression-era unemployment situation in 2020 in the U.S. as a result of the pandemic translates into less funding for many social services, whether for education (both K-12 and higher education), anti-poverty programs (the extant meager ones), or for repairing or building infrastructure such as roads. This means fewer jobs and positions in all these and many other categories of public services, agencies, and institutions generally for the public good.

Simply put, health services, restaurants, prisons, etc., were not meant to operate on the basis of interactions being six feet apart. In attempting to do so they will be a shadow of their former selves, a sort of parody of themselves.

Because of the spread of the coronavirus in close quarters such as prisons, a number of the non-violent were released, showing that perhaps these should not have been sent to prison in the first place, as they are not in other countries. Unsaid is that prison systems may not hereafter be getting the funding they had gotten before, since they do not need to hold all that many nonviolent inmates and that if they hereafter do, infection rates may skyrocket and further balloon the current spending on prisons. Taxpayers, who now have less income, are not going to be in a mood for spending on such prisons/inmates.

Still, it remains to be seen whether crime decreases overall because of the stay-at-home policies, which makes burglaries of homes more difficult for one thing. Or crime may increase because of the economic desperation of some. Most categories of crime had been decreasing the past two or three decades. The coronavirus upends the crime picture.

Assaults in the form of domestic violence have increased. Frustrations are increasing, and there are more frustrations and tensions in the U.S. in comparison with other countries which provide for their citizens. These countries ameliorate the stresses from unemployment and other factors which lead to venting frustrations on others here. Here frustrations are sometimes vent on employers who let go employees. Resources simply have not been put much in place for those in a lower income status here.

It will be a much more stressful time for those rehired, if and when they are. Under that new normal, tensions will flare, with family members at the receiving end of the violence, since many employees under these difficult conditions cannot engage in retaliation against the source, the employer, but can do so against weaker persons such as those in the family, or in the case of whites against blacks, etc. It is often pointed out that pets are at the receiving end as well by family members. Still, workplace violence may well spread simply because some employees do take out their frustrations at the decisions made by employers. Resentment against bosses in general may very well increase in time. The very insecurity of jobs is destabilizing to workers and consequently to their family. The tenuous conditions that make for both workplace violence and domestic violence are already present more so in society now that mitigation has contributed to problems.

This does not refer simply to the unemployed. It does refer to those who got a notice that they would be rehired once businesses opened up, but were not rehired. Sometimes it is not as assumed that in workplace violence it is the employer who is shot by a disgruntled employee. Fellow employees have often been the targets for particular reasons.

Moreover, police will be more reluctant to handle (and perhaps be infected in doing so) and arrest people unless they really need to do so. There were reports of police holding off on ticketing motorists during the spring of 2020. If police arrest someone just to harass, they may be risking death for themselves or their family for pulling such a stunt. It remains to be seen whether police are getting infected from arresting people, though it seems so in some reports. There may be second thoughts about closer interaction by police with suspects and guards with inmates. That, coupled with reforms arising from the protests against police brutality, will presumably modify policing practices in a more positive direction. Also positive is that some who should have never gotten arrested will not be, if from nothing else than from the anxiety about possible infection from unnecessarily handling suspects.

Crucial to this equation is that many police have families and they have to consider the possibility of transmission of the coronavirus to their families, particularly the elderly. All these matters will be weighing on the minds of the police in the near future. Those aspiring to do police work may have second thoughts about it, which careers they had eagerly embraced previously.

One thing about the risks that the coronavirus poses to most, whether police, nurses, teachers, and many others is not only the highly contagious aspect of it but that death, when death does occur, is swifter than other risks people take. A qualifier here is that some are asymptomatic and others may have gotten over the virus without knowing they had it. There are many dimensions to this virus.

Those who risk getting lung cancer by smoking may get cancer years later. Those who drink heavily may get cirrhosis of the liver years later. The latter two often belittle the possible death that many years later may result. The coronavirus risk is different. It is one that likewise might also be belittled but the consequences will be relatively very swift when COVID-19 commences, and if death occurs it will be in a matter of days or a few weeks, though some seem to linger on with the illness for a long period of time without succumbing to death very soon. Smoking and drinking alcohol are not common behaviors that all humans engage in, but interacting with others is constant (even by a five-year-old), though interaction may now be less so by many because of the coronavirus.

Thus, there is likely more anxiety about the virus though there is a good deal of bravado by many people to cover up that nervousness about getting the virus or even about dying from it. The bravado can be covered up by a nervous laughter, perhaps. One of the most important things about all this is the fact that a person that is infected can relatively quickly infect others. That is not something to joke about. There have already been instances where those who slighted the risks themselves wound up being infected and some of them died.

One thing that has been left unsaid about those who take risks is that there is in psychology what is called the personal fable. Teenagers and those in early adulthood are the ones more likely to believe in the fable, that they can take risks and will not be affected or harmed, that they are invincible, that they are different in that what happens to others will not happen to them, whether in reference to the coronavirus or speeding down the highway or getting drunk, etc. It is due to a lack of experience.

In turn much of this stems from what is termed fluid intelligence, versus crystallized intelligence. When people are younger and without experience they only have available their imagination and have to be adroit at the moment to figure out a conundrum. That is fluid intelligence, in that it is like a fluid streaming through relatively fast to deal with a novel situation because of the need to do something without the benefit of experience.

As people get older, crystallized intelligence comes more into play, where experiences crystallize and thus accumulate for them to bank on, now that they have a better idea of what to do. Those who are younger have to make do under the circumstances. Of course, neither type of intelligence disappears nor is exclusively the only one available, but one is more prominent at a point in one's life than the other for purposes of necessity, or survival if you will.

This helps explain why that early in the pandemic there were many younger people on beaches during spring break taking risks with the virus, thinking that infection happens to others but not them. Some very soon got infected and in fact apologized for their previous reckless thinking.

It must be kept in mind that those who wanted to supposedly open up the state to business, etc., were likewise reckless in regard to social distancing and some of these paid the price by getting infected as well. However, in their case they were doing what they did for political purposes, complete with Confederate flags and all, not realizing they were pawns for Trump and others. It was, though, not a matter of the personal fable (they were considerably older than teenagers) nor of fluid intelligence in their case necessarily.

Notwithstanding all this, even with a vaccine and treatment of this virus at some point, there will be a risk of infection, however minimal.

Nonetheless not all that many will want to face that risk. It is human to do all that one can to minimize the chances of dying, regardless of the level of risks, the availability of a vaccine, treatment, etc. Additionally, there are always fears and even paranoias, which will now increase exponentially.

A generalized anxiety is the worst. This is where a person cannot pinpoint a threat, but knows that one very well is lurking around somewhere. Specifically, no one can look at another and say with any certainty that that person is infected and may infect us. In other words, we don't know where the infection may come from when and if it does. Unfortunately, a much greater distrust along these lines will develop against other people.

Yet, now with so much handwashing a concomitant problem arises. All of that sanitizing of the hands can lead to a decrease in immunities, since too many of the good germs are also eliminated. The immediate benefit of constant handwashing can result in a counteraction to it, the longer term cost of becoming ill when the body no longer has resistance to some illnesses/diseases that a moderate level of handwashing would bring about. Then again, a medical person may not be able to determine what "moderate" here means and thus balance that off the cost in a decrease in immunities versus infections.

For those who cannot constantly wash their hands, there is still a risk of infection even among those who provide a service such as window/drive-up bank tellers. They provide banking services through the tubes which customers send up for a transaction. Yet the tubes and even the deposit slips and the very money itself all can carry the virus from the customer to the teller or vs. Obviously not that many people were concerned before about paper money sometimes having traces of cocaine or other drugs on it, but now the coronavirus threat is gripping many who harbor fears of touching contaminated paper money.

Money in the form of cash is thus ill-advised, though handling the credit card machines still means touching surfaces which may be contaminated. For this reason, some places provide Q-tips to use on credit card machines for entering the data for the transaction. However, in this case a person has to be extremely careful to get a new Q-tip from the container designating these as new instead from a container designating Q-tips as used. Some sort of horror might be experienced by a person making a mistake in this, akin to those who inadvertently handle biohazardous materials.

Other than on the surface of ubiquitous paper money and coins, coronavirus seems to stay for various lengths of time on surfaces, depending on what those surfaces are. Then again some purport that this is not all that much the case, but still is to some extent, and that the main form of transmission of the virus is interpersonal through respiratory droplets.

Some prominent consideration arose regarding certain jobs and positions in telemedicine ("telemed"), which was already increasing before the coronavirus, but is now increasing substantially more. This is where medical services are provided at least at first through visuals, recordings, and even live communication in real time with a health care person without it being face-to-face. There undoubtedly is a greater need for health care workers, yet telemed like other similar technological approaches applied in other careers may obviate some health care positions. This is in spite of the fact that there is a great of need for health care services particularly by the poor and others who may not have much of an internet service or a means for telemed/telehealth.

Thus it is that telemed becomes another form of inequality in health care, not much different than the less valued online courses and degrees proferred to poorer students and at a lower cost, versus the classroom face to face type for the better-off at a higher cost. In such transformations of occupations the pay for those positions decreases, relative to what the case was before. There may also still be a need which arises for more paperwork, documentation, malpractice insurance and the like, though.

Another change is that of the ER physician, who is increasingly in a more precarious position as a result of the pandemic. Namely, such a physician has been "the" presumptive doctor of the poor, who too often cannot afford to have their own doctor that they visit on a regular basis, for check-ups, and the like. But that really poses a quandary when many of the poor who have the virus have it first diagnosed and dealt with by the

ER physician and staff, when it may be too late to do much. Regardless of all the precautions taken, these health care workers cannot perfectly prevent being contaminated themselves and a number of them fall victim to the virus.

These ER persons are selfless, knowing the risks involved. They are not doing what they do to become wealthy, as some other physicians do. Still, there are some hospital ERs which have turned away a person who later tested positive for the virus. The person had gone there for fear of having the virus and thus to be diagnosed. Some of these latter patients died because they were turned away. Now hospitals have absorbed the costs of treating those with COVID-19, hoping to be compensated by the government if not by insurance which a patient may have.

The foregoing is not what occurs in some European countries with their health care for all, including foreigners visiting there, who are treated in their ER without having to pay for it. Without being concerned about receiving good health care, there is no stress about that in those countries, as there is none either about being able to afford higher education, which is also provided. There is less poverty and less crime there. It should be obvious, but it is not to many in the U.S., that such stress in this country over those and other matters breaks down the immune system, which leads to more illnesses including COVID-19 and other maladies, further confounding all of these related problems in a negative way in this society, but not in others.

Moreover, many of the above societies also have vacations which are many weeks in length for every worker. Most employers and employees here and in Europe say vacations are needed to re-charge and re-energize workers and are thus necessary. These are paid vacations, unlike the U.S. situation where there is nothing mandated to provide paid vacations for all workers and therefore to all families of said employees.

Until very recently a few states provided paid maternity leave to mothers, but that was not and is not the case for most states. Most states simply say that an employer must allow a mother (not a father as in some Scandinavian countries) up to two or three months leave, even if unpaid. Of course, many poor moms cannot afford to be without income during that time and return very soon to work.

All this illustrates the high levels of inequality in this country which lead to stressful dilemmas. This costs not only the employees in stress, his or her family suffers from the consequent tensions in myriad ways.

Inequality is also evident in the fact that some who are tested are given results sooner than others, too often indicative of discrimination: most tests results are ready in one day from a lab. Some people receive the results that soon. Trump's staff was tested daily. Apparently, the lives of everybody else are not worth it to do daily testing or much of anything else.

Meanwhile many are made to wait three days or more in receiving the results. Some had not received the results after a month. The latter was found in some largely poor rural areas of Texas, for example. Of course, this was done on the cheap there by using the National Guard in the rural areas. Instead of being taxed for more professional testing situations, those Texans had the military arrive there within only about a day's notice, not enough time to notify the townspeople, hence not many were tested. Sometimes less than ten people were tested. The "effort" was a nominal one.

The question of who gets what and when is paramount, given the urgency and anxiety to get the results once people are tested, not to mention that there is some anxiety in those who have not yet been tested. The inequality in health care knows no bounds, as is the case in other aspects of American society.

The pandemic further illuminated a dark side of hospitals, on the other hand. If medical care would be provided in the U.S., as it is in a number of European countries and elsewhere, on a preventive basis, that would be better for the populace as a whole than relying on the profits from elective services here. Elective surgeries, often referred to as non-essential surgeries, were the profitable mainstays of hospitals. However much that health care workers heroically struggled to save the lives of patients, the latter were not very profitable for the hospitals.

Now many realized how it is after all that hospitals generally are in a lucrative business. So much so is this that there are hospital closings if they are not profitable as a business, regardless of the need for health care in a given community. At that point the ill will have to travel perhaps thirty miles or more to the nearest hospital. In a word, the needed health care was not profitable enough, so they closed. This can be referred to as a hospital desert, with a community left stranded without a hospital. This is no different than food deserts in poor communities, including in large cities, where a poor area is not deemed profitable enough for a major supermarkets and there is a dearth of groceries. All this is what too many blacks, Latinos, and poor whites face more than others.

In a word, society found out that elective surgeries eclipse the needed medical services for all in the U.S. Instead society now may be paying for all the necessary health care being done for the COVID-19 patients, many of them unable to pay, being as they are of low income or no income in the case of the unemployed. Of course, those of lower income are more likely to have underlying health issues to begin with and thus their immune system not withstand the coronavirus. They had not treated the underlying health problems because they did not have health insurance or it was inadequate, in contrast to better-off persons with good health care and therefore better immunities to illness.

Moreover, it seems that the virus can return and re-infect a person, although there are some things unclear about this. The meaning of getting well might well undergo further qualifications. This complicates the confidence some have placed in a cure: there may not be much of a cure in the foreseeable future. Health care workers may become overwhelmed more than they are now, not the least of reasons being that the poor in the U.S. or elsewhere in the world may see skyrocketing infections. These questions remain rather unanswered now but will be answered as time goes by.

Thus it is that aspiring medical students have second thoughts about their plans, while medical students and graduates from usually poorer foreign countries come to the U.S., as has occurred significantly with physicians and nurses. Nurses have been coming to the U.S. for at least forty years from the Philippines, for example, since the pay is very low in their country. They are only doing what they think is right and are as qualified as anyone else in the medical world or may train to be certified as such. This is called a brain drain by the country of origin whereby the country invests in these students in their K-12 and collegiate education and then sees them coming to the U.S. Given the problems health care workers have encountered in caring for COVID-19 patients, there will probably be an increase in health care workers from other countries to the U.S. while there is more uncertainty about the pipeline here given the questions about medical careers.

Not only that, the number of health care workers of color are increasing because their populations are increasing in the U.S. All of the above became easy to see in newscasts about COVID-19. That is one of the reasons whites are alarmed and in their protests proclaim and chant "We will not be replaced." They fear replacement by those of color, particularly in socioeconomic terms. The replacement will definitely accelerate, given the reality of demographics. For example, older white males are the more politically likely to follow Trump, and they are declining in population. The younger followers of Bernie Sanders have been gaining ground, on the other hand.

Another facet of telemed and working from home and teleconferencing is the qualitative aspect of that work that is relatively lacking and is known as body language. This is also referred to as nonverbal communication. This is of importance because in social services in particular the nonverbal is an integral part of the interactive process, and that cannot be gauged just by looking at talking heads. The body may be something that contradicts what a person verbally articulates.

Psychologists and counselors need to see the entire person if they are to assist in therapy, especially now that anxieties and fears are increasing due to the virus and potential death from it. The anxious staff at nursing homes are increasingly admonished not to hug the elderly residents, lest they infect them or vs. That is because many who have the coronavirus are asymptomatic yet contagious.

The solace one gets from hugging is declining, though hugging is needed now more than ever with the uncertainties throughout society. The gesture of hugging grandma becomes suspect, not the least of reasons being that infecting the elderly can be more so fatal for them than someone hugging and infecting a younger person.

Even if this lack of hugging is temporary, with the upcoming availability of a vaccine and treatment, family members would not want to risk grandpa at the nursing home being infected by a staff member or health care provider. Apparently, Dr. Hug (Leo Buscaglia) will be largely forgotten in time. There will be some in the near future who will dwell on the nostalgia of his presentations and writings. That he may come to be seen as quaint is unfortunate. Health concerns may very well trump Dr. Hug.

Because hugging is, otherwise than in regard to the coronavirus, very positive, it must be reiterated as to why that is the case. Specifically, there are health benefits from hugging, such as the healthy electro-chemical discharge that occurs from someone touching another. Even premature babies in incubators benefit and the elderly had been benefitting from touching. The neurotransmitters in the brain produced beneficial outcomes to a person being hugged, unless a person did not like the person hugging him or her. It is a sad commentary that much of this about hugging and touching may be tossed to the wayside now.

Those in occupations such as elementary school teaching will think twice about hugging their students, regardless of the health benefits psychologically and physiologically. Some children were getting their hugs only or primarily from their teachers, what with the stresses and problems many parents face. Nonetheless and not surprisingly school districts will develop policies, guidelines, prohibitions, etc., about these interactions.

At the least, parents might raise eyebrows when a teacher hugs their child, or even if the child hugs the teacher as some children are wont to do. It can be a simple pat on the shoulder, common before the coronavirus, that can trigger a lawsuit against a district if a teacher infects a student when and if there are policies prohibiting any physical interaction. That could cost school districts money, especially if a death is thought to have been the consequence from touching. Ultimately, cameras might be installed in the classroom, as they are around some buildings. That would be an added cost to school districts but perhaps deemed necessary by school districts, affecting the economy/funding of education.

All this does not negate the fact that teachers work quite closely with students, especially younger children, whether hugging or not. Since parents are not in the classroom all day, it is conceivable that parents will start asking their children if the teacher touched them on the head, shoulders, or (anathema) hugged them during the school day. Parents are concerned not only with a teacher or staff member infecting their child but also with that child consequently infecting others in the family, particularly elderly grandparents.

Nevertheless, students touch each other during the day, if nothing else than just to get one's attention, among other things. They will be in physical contact with each other on the playground, during contact sports, and so forth. Then there is the fact that they will touch objects that others touched, and not only doorknobs. The question arises of what will become of playballs they throw to each other, toys they play with, gym equipment, even the rails ballet students hold onto. The economic cost of sanitizing all these surfaces is unimaginable at this point.

Everything cannot be sanitized all the time. The only hope is that the research was not all that accurate about the virus active on a number of substances for various lengths of time, depending on what the substances are. If seems that research on contamination of objects is accurate even if to some extent, and sanitizing still plays a major role in regard to the coronavirus, witnessed by grocery stores continuously sanitizing all their carts for months on end.

In other words, institutional liability particularly in the monetary sense may become a major issue. Currently, for example, there are institutions such as prisons where contagiousness is essentially prevalent in comparison to other settings, yet not many people have taken to task the liability and responsibility prisons have in their overcrowding in regard to this pandemic. Apparently, not many in society care about inmates and their problems, whether it is violence therein, rapes, or brutality by guards, not to mention myriad violations of the constitutional rights of inmates. Concern increases only when prison staff are infected, as many are now.

As for economic circumstances in other countries, especially the poorer ones, all this in reference to the societal changes from the coronavirus is unexplored terrain. In poor countries many do not have much education and thus cannot know the details/nuances about infection and contamination. Many of them are at the level the U.S. was previously: not believing much about viruses and germs and dismissing what they cannot see, and therefore understandably scoffing at such. Furthermore, a vaccine and treatment will not reach the poor in these countries to a great extent. At this point they haven't tested much.

Much the same can be said about testing for HIV, the virus causing AIDS. Specifically, a person can test negative for HIV today but contract it tomorrow, or thereafter. The person would have the impression that he or she is simply negative, while a test for it later might find him or her testing positive. This testing scenario is similar to that of the coronavirus. Furthermore, both viruses can be fatal. In that sense this is unlike testing for other diseases which are not fatal, making the testing for the coronavirus and HIV so crucial.

Yet there has not been as much testing for some of these viruses as there should be. Were there to be very extensive testing in the U.S., that does not mean that would the case for the rest of the world. Not only that, the social aspects of testing to a large extent would mean in time there would be discrimination, ostracism and disdain for those who had not yet tested for the coronavirus. In those situations, simply put, those who had not been tested likely would not reveal that to others.

In the purely economic sense, the billions who are poor in the world cannot focus on their health every day, except for those already quite ill. Subsistence makes them desperate for income. In India some sell cardboards they find or canisters they come across. Some sell produce in open-air markets devoid of sanitation. In Mexico some on highways sell goat cheese, snake skins, even small live animals such as birds and fawns to passers-by. In crossing the border into Mexico one encounters the ubiquitous beggars and the sellers of fake jewelry, or children begging to wash one's car or windows, albeit with dirty water. Sometimes they offer for income to watch a car for a tourist while the latter parks it to shop or dine somewhere.

Even in the U.S. some desperate for income will work in high-risk occupations. One of those is that of workers who repair roads and in doing so breathe carcinogenic tar all day. A person cannot mention that to them without the worker saying there is nothing else and besides that they cannot see the cancer they will contract in a number of years, if they contract it. Viruses likewise cannot be seen and can thereby be dismissed. Workers need money this very day.

Certainly, the better-off countries have an obligation to assist the poorer ones whether in regard to the coronavirus now in the poor countries or in other matters. In a word, the better-off countries generally became so at the expense of the poorer ones, such as Belgium at the expense of the Congo as just one example. Belgium owes much to the Congo from which the former extracted the resources from the Congo, such as so much gold (which cost the lives of Africans) that it lines many buildings in Belgium. Payback is referred to as reparations, similar to blacks in the U.S. demanding reparations from whites due to how slavery benefited whites in general. It can be framed as a matter of the eventual white privilege which even poor whites have to an extent. Alternatively, even wealthy blacks still on the other hand suffer from racism.

Reparations were paid out from the U.S. government to the Japanese who were forced onto concentration camps in Arizona during World War II. Germany paid reparations to Jews who suffered from that country's policies during World War II also. By that standard, the U.S. owes trillions to Iraq, Afghanistan, Vietnam and many other countries, including in Latin America (over twenty-one invasions of Latin American countries by the U.S.), such as in Nicaragua, Cuba, Mexico and elsewhere.

If not reparations, a prominent general put a different lens on this of what would have been the alternative. He said the U.S. would have been convicted of war crimes if it had lost World War II because of the wanton destruction, including the unnecessary nuclear bombings of civilians in Japan.

Even Prince Harry from the British royalty admitted lately that Britain will have to confront its colonialist past, as the U.S. is doing about its explorers, presidents, and other leaders here. Thus it is that many in the U.S. are bringing down racist monuments and further pursuing reparations, among other things.

Money-wise, throughout the world important health care issues arise from the lack of funding for enough testing for the virus, ventilators, proper masks, etc. Yet billions of dollars are instead shoveled into the war machine, much of it fraudulently spent with no accountability.

On the contrary, the lack of concern for others is palpable in this society. It is in fact thoroughgoing in the very violence officially and unofficially from the founding of the country to wrest the land from Native Americans. The latter are at the bottom of American society, with many in reservations where they live poverty-stricken. They have been in Depression-era levels of unemployment for decades. The policy of the U.S. government originally for them was that of genocide. Hitler adopted his ideas of genocide from and praised the U.S. for the efficiency of the starvation and extermination of Native Americans. He also studied and admired the American practice in the first half of the 1900s of sterilization of "undesirables." He learned from the U.S. and applied it in the Holocaust.

The violence continued apace against blacks as slaves, with the very first intimations of policing in the U.S. being the slave patrols who were on the lookout to retrieve runaway slaves back to their slave masters. Then it continued against Latinos, in particular against Chicanos in Texas by the Texas Rangers officially even, in many instances, to kill brown people as at Porvenir, Texas and steal the land from them in the Valley of Texas and elsewhere. The Rangers were deemed the official KKK against Chicanos. Yet a professional baseball team was named after them, regardless (as glaringly as the Redskins got their moniker). Undoubtedly, Chicanos root for the Texas Rangers baseball team, not knowing the historical roots of the Rangers.

In fact, violence was nothing new and in fact was extolled in many ways by Trump himself. He called for his gun-toting followers and others to "Liberate" the state, and they duly appeared at state capitols to do so. Trump even gratuitously mentioned at the time, without any reason to do so, the Second Amendment about bearing arms. Anyone else inciting others with such inflammatory language would be investigated for promoting terrorism. In other words, he wanted to salve his anxiety for saving his cherished economic system to regain, at any cost, the ground the economy had lost (a lost cause), whether people got infected in the process and died or not. Again, it is no surprise that Martin Luther King highlighted the pervasive violence the U.S. promotes here and in the world.

The first thing some developed countries might think, though, is what is in it for them, and perhaps how they could profit from assisting others. The similarity to the ER at a hospital arises, in that before there may not at first sight be a benefit for the hospital to take those who arrive at its door, and there are many examples of they instead sending a person to another hospital's ER when that person does not have health insurance. That is called patient dumping. However, it would cost society to have someone with the coronavirus be refused somewhere, and in the process of going elsewhere or nowhere for help, that person might infect others.

In that sense American society does what it does to help some because too often it is ultimately in society's benefit to assist. Likewise the richer countries need to help those countries not doing well, particularly in regard to the virus, since it might ultimately cost the richer ones in infections from the lesser developed countries and even in deaths, what with the ease of travel from one place to another. It is in the interest of everyone to assist each other, the Christian way supposedly, if nothing else than for some to save their own skin (future monies and lives).

Still, many of those unemployed during the closings of businesses had little or no income coming into the household, yet in farm fields the produce was left to rot (as indicated previously, cattle have been slaughtered, wheat burned and milk poured down the gutters when the commodity prices aren't "right" for ranchers and farmers) though people were hungry, including many children. With schools closed, milk companies lost the lucrative school district as customers, though some of the milk was not that successfully diverted to groceries.

Some food giveaways from food pantries sprouted at various times during the pandemic, but there could have been much more done in a supposedly Christian country which instead expects payment for most anything. Thousands of churches would need to collect thousands of dollars more each week as charity to supplant, not just to supplement, government assistance to the poor by those who say that churches should be the ones helping people, and that does not happen. The poor mostly fend for themselves, while the wealthy and the corporations easily receive corporate welfare, all the while feigning that they have succeeded on their own. Thus it is that some categories of people with less resources become more vulnerable to the coronavirus than others.

Yet the media tugs at the heart strings when, without fail every Thanksgiving, they show the poor given one meal in some large hall for the year. That's it. It is the first item in the local news usually, so proud that the media and the community are about this showing of magnanimity, when in the grand scheme of things in the economy this is essentially inconsequential.

Whatever happens, undoubtedly the economy in trouble in this society will affect the economies of other countries. The repercussions are bidirectional. The economies in trouble elsewhere will affect the U.S. as well. Interdependence among countries ensures it, not only in the economic sense but also in regard to infections and deaths. Isolationism is defunct. Simply put, because of our policies the chickens have come home to roost, a saying that Ward Churchill repeated after 9-11 at great cost to him.

Those in political office cite a so-called pent-up demand occurring in the "opening up" of the economy. Pent-up demands do not necessarily lead to pent-buying. Whatever people might want is not going to be matched by their ability to pay for it, what with many getting lower paying jobs than they had before (complete with uncompensated speed up demanded of those still at a workplace to make up for those the boss downsized), if they still have a job. Many will not have anything at all anymore.

The pent-up demands are not going to be fulfilled by those who have a decent but unsteady job, as workers now feel uneasy about prospects for long-term employment. More therefore will be risk-averse about purchasing expensive items such as houses and cars, not to mention other types of purchases. There is a greater likelihood of more frugality and less of careless abandon and risk, particularly with a family in tow.

The stimulus checks have not made a decisive difference. Alaska has been sending checks to its citizens on a regular basis as has the country of Norway. A lot more stimulus is needed.

Obviously if a pent-up demand developed for luxury cars by many in the general population, it does not mean therefore that they will buy them. A Rolls Royce bought by the rich, whose wealth skyrocketed during the pandemic, is a more likely scenario, while others will settle for a Chevy or no car at all.

What might not get a boost from the pandemic is public transportation, for the simple reason that such passengers are in close quarters with fellow travelers, and thus more conducive to acquiring the contagious virus. With high levels of unemployment there may be a need for more public transportation which may have been met in pre-pandemic times, but the risk of infection in crowded modes of public transportation seems to such ridership now a rather moot point.

All this means as well that of those who do have a job, tensions may flare more than before the pandemic with so much uncertainty now over major concerns. Uncertainties over employment and/or the possibility of getting infected weigh heavily on millions of people throughout the U.S. and the world.

Chapter 7

Politics

The political refers to power, the capacity to do things, which does not necessarily correlate with being rational about anything that is done. Most of political power is based on money. (Money talks….) The pandemic has forced the hand of the political world in countless and very crucial ways.

From the standpoint of political sociology, all things strictly political will change because of the coronavirus. Then again nothing is strictly political because the electioneering affects all other realms. Already in the spring of 2020 President Trump was having daily press conferences which were basically political (for re-election purposes) in substance but touted as updates on the coronavirus. Nevertheless, he abandoned the daily briefings in short order when they became a liability and were no longer helping his political stock and image.

Early on he affirmed that the virus was under control and made claims that minimized it. There are what sociologists since the days of theorist Thorstein Veblen call vested interests (which are primarily monetary). In Trump's case his vested interest was his candidacy, which was on the line in the upcoming presidential election in only a matter of months since the coronavirus contagion. He engaged in grandstanding about supposedly superlative accomplishments of his administration to mitigate the loss of many thousands of lives. Basically, he was more concerned, as he always has been, with Business as usual with a capital B, as well as about his personal optics and the optics of the stock market (greed is good, according to the market) and the economy.

It is clear that because of his political anxieties about his political image, what he needed to do in the early stages of the pandemic in the U.S. he failed to do. He was warned about the pandemic, while later he claimed he was not. In a word his basic concern was saving the profit-driven but tottering economy, not the COVID-19 deaths. That became clear when by early June 2020 he held no press conferences on the virus which he had previously held every day. He did hold rallies, though, for the upcoming election after he abandoned the briefings.

Nevertheless, the economy was shattered anyway, but now with many thousands of people dying, too. Subsequently his political image was battered as well. The obvious physical anguish in his visage betrayed his policies/actions. Such nonverbal communication of his says volumes, but very few commentators even mention the obvious. The psychologists and others are nowhere to be found to point it out.

There is some similarity in his situation to that which George W. Bush encountered after 9-11. At the time Bush in his anxiety exhorted people to go shopping to save the system. Many did and got into debt from following Bush's exhortations to bolster the economy. The nexus between 9-11 and the economy did not affect everyone in society than the way that the pervasive anxiety over the coronavirus does now, though. 9-11 did not lead to the shutting down of the economy and various institutions (schools, churches, etc.) for months as in the case of the coronavirus. The difference is qualitative and quantitive.

Bush, though, emphasized shopping (which profited businesses) since it is an activity that those who are upper class as well as those who are lower class can engage in, as if the two classes were equal in their shopping or anything else. However, the lower class will, like anybody else, be treated courteously and with dignity while shopping, one of the few instances they will be. Not only that, shopping is purportedly a situation where the upper class and lower class can buy some of the same products, again as if they were equal. Bush sought to prop up the temporarily faltering economy from 9-11 and to distract the shoppers from the intelligence failures leading to 9-11.

Bush was supposedly addressing terrorism. Yet his administration and that of other presidents has provided sanctuary in the U.S. for those wanted for terrorism in El Salvador, Venezuela, and Cuba, to mention a few countries. Such terrorism has killed many throughout the world, yet the terrorists live safely in the U.S., particularly in Florida. These major transgressions of the U.S. government go unchecked and the discussions of terrorism are essentially hypocritical. It should be no surprise that our claims of caring about people here in this country and elsewhere in regard to the coronavirus are similarly hypocritical.

There are other situations in society where it seems that all classes, all people, can mingle as if all are equal, such as at a pro football game. This is particularly so if they are "equally" rooting for the same team and, for example, the upper and lower class give each other high fives during the game. The high fives may be less common now with the coronavirus. Another similar example of purported equality among people regardless of class and race is at church. Martin Luther King had something to say about that. He critiqued the Sunday church hour as the most segregated in American society.

As for major transgressions by corporations in the U.S., Nancy Pelosi was caught nervously blinking her eyes nonstop when filmed after she caved to corporations who threatened chaos because of the 2008 economy collapsing. She was present at the public announcement of Congress shoring up the corporations and thus the economy through bailouts from taxpayer money. She may not do that to shore up our health care system, unless it would involve corporate health care.

Such a salvaging job cannot be quite done anymore with the much more extensive devastation from the coronavirus. The result is the ongoing economic train wreck. Were it not for the gargantuan squandering of our blood and treasure and decades of profiteering by corporations we would be a healthier society with more resources, as is the case with many other nations that more wisely did what they did. Now they have some very positive results to show for their policies and approaches to problems and are better off for it monetarily and in other aspects. Meanwhile the coronavirus has raged on here, even as apologists for our economic system minimize it.

So many changes have transpired as a result of the coronavirus. Another example not often acknowledged are the low gasoline prices. These were a consequence of the steep decline in travel in the U.S., making oil abundant and low-priced for those who did travel particularly by motor vehicle. Those motorists got a taste of what it was like to pay much less for gas, about $1.50 a gallon at one point, and they now realize that a world of low gas prices is possible, but it has been artificially inflated for the profiteering oil companies. Not only do oil companies profit, so do the superfluous salespersons of gas guzzlers, and others who cost society in innumerable ways, including our health (from those who pollute the air, etc.).

Said motorists, and everyone else, have had their eyes opened and are not happy campers about the deceptions that now cost them money, money which they could have allocated to their families instead, perhaps for much needed vacations which would boost their immune systems from the relief of stresses at work. There is a possibility that such circumstances would have fortified our society better to confront the virus, health-wise. This greater fortification would have benefitted those whose immune system is currently compromised. This is important because it appears that people's immune systems are not as strong as had been assumed when the coronavirus hit, and that is a result of deficient health care.

No matter how much of the hourglass looks horrific, Trump proclaimed the smaller part of it that was sunny, again with an upcoming election in mind. He intimidated reporters such that they didn't take him too much to task. Instead reporters railed against his personality, as the media is wont to do and look at the micro, the human interest aspects, instead of extensively investigating the macro economic impact of his failures on society. To put it more exactly, the economic failures are very much structural anyway and not all that strictly under his control. Very questionable is how many journalists would want to look at their own media conglomerate, that is.

How Trump looks, optics, is the number one thing to him, whether in relation to the coronavirus or the protests. Hence, at one point he hurriedly created a photo-op at a church across the street right after peaceful protestors were tear-gassed to make room for him crossing the street.

Still, the future will be one where political candidates as contenders will have to address the previous call by Bernie Sanders for comprehensive health care for all, given what the coronavirus has wrought. The pandemic occurred after Bernie's candidacy and thus candidates did not have to confront much anymore his issues about health care, until now again. There are, though, some candidates who state that the extensive military waste and the pork will need to be dealt with if the U.S. is to succeed in providing health care, as other countries have.

More funding, it is evident, will need to be diverted therefore to health care and education and elsewhere. That increase in funding could come from a decrease in the funding of police departments. Funding of the police too often is outsized. This is what is meant by defunding the police. Safety does not result from funding extensive police brutality and the militarization of the police (including wartime weapons that the military dumped on the police departments for a pretty penny), just as safety does not result from wasted monies on fraudulent military expenditures. Aggression by police and abuse create problems. Education and health care (needed more now because of the virus) are positive and constructive.

As to allocations for education, taxes will need to be diverted from the obscene military funding to pay teachers their combat pay, as it is called, as one example because of the new health risks of the occupation. It will become necessary to entice more college students into the teaching profession, if that can even be easily done given the new coronavirus scenarios in education. This is similar to the enticements the military offers to young people to enlist them, the enlistment bonuses, where otherwise they would not be interested in an occupation where they might get killed, as 7,000 were in Afghanistan and Iraq, not to mention many more thousands we killed in those countries when we invaded them for purposes of oil and gas profits.

However, it is better to entice people into a career in education rather than one in training to be a professional killer. This writer had been in the military for several years and in education for a lifetime and the contrasts were stark, in the macro and any other sense. The money wasted in illegal military ventures needs to be diverted or redirected to education and health care, among other more positive things in society, as it has been in other societies.

Most who enlist in the military do so anyway for the education benefits and health care they are to receive. That is a roundabout way of getting an education and health care, while perhaps getting killed in war or injured in the process. We hurriedly send the lower income enlistees out there but do not provide (VA) much when they return. Many presidents and many in Congress send them out there to die in combat, but not their own selves or their own sons and daughters. Bush did not his military age daughters.

There will evolve a clamor for higher taxes on the wealthy, as some of the wealthy themselves promulgate. The wealthy might mute their voice in public in the future, lest they further raise the ire of the non-wealthy. The clamor of those who strive to work for a living wage will grow as it has not before. As a matter of fact, surveys had already indicated that socialism was held at a higher regard by a greater percent of the American electorate than was previously the case and particularly so by younger Americans.

The ideology of capitalism slid. This happens when people see that, for example, the income of billionaires increased greatly during the pandemic, in contrast to everyone else. The coronavirus ramifications such as unemployment, more precarious employment, etc., have contributed to many thinking that they cannot afford nor need much "stuff" after all, which leads to a speedier collapse of the economic system.

As a matter of fact, many had in recent history been in jobs which were referred to as contingent work. Contingent means that something depends on something else. In this case it means that jobs depend on whatever the bosses want and that employees don't have much say or choice in the matter anymore, if they ever did much. Therefore, the types of jobs which were increasing recently quite rapidly were contingent types, such as part-time, temporary, self-employed, and contract work. The ramifications of the coronavirus will accelerate an increase in the contingent category of employment.

One question will still remain as always. Some surveys show, just like some billionaires themselves say, that taxes should go up in order to provide more and better services. Respondents state that they don't mind if their taxes increase if they know if it is for good purposes. The problem with income taxes, though, is that those taxed do not know where their money is being allocated, and it often is for wasteful purposes that benefit only some at the expense of the vast majority.

There are those who, because of their shattered jobs and economy, will be earning less and will not be too excited about their low income being taxed for waste. Many of those earning lower incomes would prefer better and more affordable health care and education from higher taxes on the wealthy. It is questionable that the exclamation by some candidates that they will not raise taxes will resonate with the electorate as it had before. That exclamation has not carried much weight with Europeans and others who preferred the benefits that higher taxes brought than the costs. They saw what they got in return in their societies such as less crime, greater longevity, less poverty, more free education at the collegiate level, the provision of free or very low-cost day care, and other pluses.

Of course, many in Congress do not want the above type of free health care for all which in fact the members of Congress have for themselves. They keep that type of health care for themselves and do not abandon it, though they of all people could afford to pay for their own health care out of their own pocket. However, they don't want their own constituents to have it and thus society be taxed for it, as is the case with Europeans who are fine with the taxation because they are fine with the outcomes from it.

In sum, hypocrisy reigns supreme among those in Congress and some presidents: they send others to die in combat but not their own selves and their offspring. They also have excellent health care provisions which most of them do not want provided for others. Those who contract COVID-19 should confront Congress.

Perhaps we will perceive what the outsized military expenditures have done to our society. The military power can be likened to photos of a homeowner standing with a rifle on top of the rubble caused by a hurricane. The person has the weapon to supposedly protect the useless rubble, with nothing left to save or protect, but the pretense of doing so: just the mere semblance of doing so is all that is left, empty posturing.

Perhaps we likewise have the expensive military weapons to supposedly protect the useless rubble of an economy devastated now by the coronavirus, not to mention whatever there was of democracy before, now shredded as well. Questionable itself is our very claim of democracy, since Saudi Arabia never has been one, yet we ply that country with weaponry. They do have oil. Crass monetary considerations prevail in American history, as the shroud has now fallen off of such crassness because of the ramifications from the coronavirus.

In other words, there may not be anything left to protect anymore, just an empty gesture. Essentially nothing of value is left after military expenditures have squandered whatever chance we might have had to have a stronger economy of value for all.

The devastation is that of an entrenched inequality in health care, education, the economy, and so forth. Even black businesses before the virus were too often on the edge and the coronavirus pushed many of them off the precipice. The great majority of businesses are small business, with about one third closing down within three years while half do so within just five years, sprouting here and there and gone relatively soon thereafter.

The inequality in another institution, the criminal justice system, is so entrenched that the infection and death rates from the virus are skyrocketing among those incarcerated. The gauge of equality or the lack thereof in a given society is often cited in the manner the society treats the inmates in prison. At this rate, American society apparently does not care to any significant extent about the conditions in prisons. Not to unnecessarily focus on the Bible, but even there many Christians do not practice what they were commanded, to do for the least of us. That sure is not the highlight of our society.

It would not be surprising therefore to hear some people wish that those in prison die from COVID-19. Currently, being jailed and imprisoned is becoming in reality a possible death sentence. That is a form of cruel and unusual punishment which is constitutionally illegal, which is why some have been released to mitigate the coronavirus raging there and possible deaths (of both inmates and prison staff). The prisoners were not all sentenced there for murder and violent offenses, but society may be guilty of murdering, in this sense, many inmates in keeping the nonviolent ones there for that very outcome. Vaccines, treatment and testing of the coronavirus will not be a priority there. Not realized is that the problems inmates face while in prison eventually become our problems, one way or another. The vast majority are released back into society, back into the same hopeless circumstances, but now harboring pent-up feelings about their ordeals there.

They are not going to be happy campers when released, with over half returning to prison within a few years after release (the rate of return is referred to as recidivism). They will be more bitter at the society that sent them there, given that a number of them were innocent after all, or sentenced for drug offenses. Inmates often faced beatings and rapes there. They did not have much going for them before prison, nor will they after. Disproportionately they are black and Latino, with the rest poor whites, almost all of them having little education. Society mistakenly thought it closed a chapter by consigning them to those hell holes. Society will bear the consequences, the price will be paid for sending them there, and not only in more virus infections on the outside of prison walls when released.

Of violent offenses, particularly murder, almost all of these are committed in the heat of the moment from frustrations, tensions, and palpable inequality in society. European societies which have lower rates of violent crime, including murder, have fewer tensions, given that they don't have much of a reason to be stressed out and feeling the tension of a high rate of inequality. There is more equality there. Very significantly, because many provide free health care, free higher education, have less poverty, free day care, among other things, there is no reason for people there to be mortified about things and lash out at others, which is what violence is and manifested here.

The media here focus on premeditated murders, what are referred to as cold-blooded killings. These types are rare. More likely what happens in murders is that a person gets upset at another person on the spot, at a bar perhaps, or on the highway, etc., with emotions running high. The availability of a gun means he or she will reach for it to quickly resolve some dispute there or in a family setting or out of stress and the heat of the moment, emotions, etc. The media does not focus on all these situations, which constitute the great majority of murders, because then the media might have to discuss how to resolve the frustrations we have here: by doing what European societies do to ease problems in society. That means funding positive programs and increased taxation.

Now we have the coronavirus threat as an added layer of stress in this society in addition to the other sources of stress. Indeed, the stress in regard to the coronavirus is there in European societies, but not the other aforementioned tensions that we in our society have but do not alleviate. The Japanese likewise are not stressed out about crime. So much so is this the case that it is not unusual for their children to walk to school and even commute on the subway to get to school without their parents.

So, those which could be called "hot-blooded killings" will not be called that or discussed at length. If we did look at the sources of tension we would have to admit that we should address those sources, which cost society in money and lives. In spite of all this, the media sells the calculated cold-blooded murders (no emotions, solely an elaborate plan to kill someone).

All the entrenched inequality in health care and other institutions is now laid bare more than before as a result of the coronavirus. The urgency is arising to fix all this in a day, but that is not very feasible. Much of the previous repair work consisted of palliatives, meant to squelch the uproars, as was the case after the Los Angeles uprising of 1992. Even the token programs to ameliorate conditions in the city were soon abandoned after things quieted down, once the uprising subsided. It remains to be seen what follows in the wake of recent protests over police brutality against blacks and others. Currently blacks face higher rates of unemployment, more coronavirus infections, and a higher rate of killings by police than other segments of the population, a triple whammy.

As just one example of how society recently witnessed the fact that policing is systemically racist was in the treatment of protestors. Much has been filmed and documented on the attacks by police and others against those peacefully protesting the killings of blacks. Examples follow: whites themselves saw what police officers (not the "one bad apple" appellation) did not only to George Floyd; there were six police who violently pulled two Morehouse college students from their car who were doing nothing against the police; the attack by Austin police against a black Texas State University student (which belies the liberal designation of Austin) causing him brain damage and also injured a pregnant woman; the four police who beat up a cyclist who simply was going too slow in front of them; law enforcement attacking peaceful protestors in front of the White House so Trump could have his photo op; the large number of police who passed by the bleeding 75 year old who was pushed to the pavement by police; the large number of police (actually filmed) slashing tires of protestors and reporters; the New Jersey corrections officer and another mocking the death of Floyd, the instances of police cars plowing into protestors, and so forth, and these were only some of the ones filmed.

We would not have known what police did if not filmed (some police, before they recently attacked protestors turned off their body cameras). The vast majority of police attacking people have not been filmed throughout American history.

For those not clear about black lives not mattering (because they have not in policing, health care, education, etc.), even Mitt Romney now said that Black Lives Matter. That black lives do not matter to police, is seen by Temple, Texas, police for months not releasing the video of a black man being shot in the head by a police officer. This police officer was Latino. People of color can take on the ethos of whites as that of their own, just as many slaves did. Hiring more police of color thus is not a complete answer by any means to brutality against those of color.

Just how much uncertainty there is now of what has transpired in the history of policing and people of color was seen in the simple fact that the PD Live TV show was cancelled after a black man was filmed who died after saying he could not breathe while in custody and the video of it was destroyed. The Cops TV show was also cancelled. The level-headed portrayal of police in those shows is caput, with police brutality edited out and not selected for showing. In a matter of a few days both shows disappeared from TV. The exponential ramifications of the coronavirus are legend.

Due to uncertainties from the virus, unsurprisingly, purchases of smaller homes and cars are in tune with a more cautious and uncertain economic situation concerning people's jobs. However, many of those who can afford to buy bigger homes will do so in the interest of social distancing and not simply because some can afford to do so. Sure, the bigger vehicles, particularly the Hummer (named after the military

Humvee), coincided with the American bravado over Iraqis, before. Iraqis were incorrectly insinuated by Bush as causing 9/11, and thousands of them died in the illegal invasion and occupation by the U.S., along with thousands of American soldiers.

A similar type of bravado comes from those who deride and dismiss the risks of the coronavirus. Success in the economy is more important to these types than preventing deaths from the virus, just like victory (which never occurred) in the Middle East was more important to the U.S. and Britain at the time than the hundreds of thousands of consequent gruesome deaths for oil, though it all came to naught, nothing gained after all, just losses in blood and treasure for millions of people affected one way or another.

In the same vein, President Johnson once admitted in private that the Vietnam War was worthless for him. He only felt shame were he to be the first president to lose a war, and lose the war he did, along with Nixon. Even at that time resources squandered for Vietnam could have been used for health care and other positive things. Defunding of the Vietnam War would have meant resources diverted from the war to positive things, similar to the concept of defunding of the police today.

Interestingly, and very tragically, police departments in the U.S. have gotten military hardware. That is added to the fact that too many combat veterans who killed others in Iraq and Afghanistan are now police shooting people here, trigger-happy as they were in the Middle East with deadly consequences for people there. Now we see the results here, particularly against blacks. Racist terms were used by combat soldiers for people there as well, such as sand niggers and ragheads, just as they had racist terms for the Vietnamese as gooks, etc.

Moreover, the general directing the war there, Westmoreland, stated in racist terms that Asians did not value life as Americans did, goading American soldiers to slaughter them. Before him, Secretary of State Kissinger indicated that the people of Chile were inferior in their thinking. The racism from the top of society is not new, except to those who do not read much. Social Darwinism which postulates that some people are more fit and superior to others has been around for over 100 years, with Britain and the U.S. the main subscribers to such thought.

Also, in reference to racism and classism in a political sense in the U.S. with this most serious of viruses, it remains to be seen what category of class gets ventilators, vaccines and treatment when these become available, even who gets quality masks and gloves. Everybody will not get these equally. With what the history of health care indicates, it should not be difficult to discern who gets what. In fact this has already been seen with the poorer and those of color suffering more than better-off whites. Testing for the virus is already patently racist, with whites more likely than blacks and Latinos being tested. Perhaps, as has been noted by many writers recently, treatment should be given according to socioeconomic need instead of a fat pocketbook.

Emergency rooms are examples where treatment is supposedly allocated according to need. Unsaid about this is that this is done not out of the goodness of society's collective heart but because you cannot have someone walking around bleeding in the community or dying on the sidewalk or someone walking around infecting other people (in the case of the coronavirus). The care in the ER is meant to therefore obviate bigger problems. If it were the case as it is in much of Europe of genuine concern for others there would be preventive health care, instead of patching up others for the moment after the fact.

Those elected to the higher offices in the country are mostly from the aforementioned upper classes and attorneys, not health care providers. Trump's background is from the financial class of real estate moguls. Though he has repeated that he is not a medical doctor, he nevertheless has frequently trumped medical experts and has directly kept them from answering questions from the media about the coronavirus. He answers the questions about the virus.

This is unconscionable. Real estate is his background, not medicine. Yet he gives medical recommendations even about what drug to take to counter the virus, contradicting medical experts. He initially stated that those afflicted with the virus miraculously would be down to zero. Basically, Trump during the pandemic pandered to his political base, who duly picked up what he touted. He very well knew that they would.

By the summer of 2020 the president was casting aspersions on Dr. Fauci, the chief immunologist on the coronavirus task force. Trump savaged him when he was no longer expedient for furthering Trump's view of saving the economic system. The president then relented.

With the expanding pandemic, the need is apparent for greater international cooperation than there has been. Whether that need determines what political leaders do is another thing, witnessed by the bloody invasions and assaults by the U.S. of Afghanistan, Iraq, Syria, Libya, Vietnam and many other countries. All this is in addition to the history of the U.S. being one of violence against others internationally, and violence within the country.

For the most part American students are not taught and thus know next to nothing about even where Iraq and Afghanistan are on a map, all the while that thousands of Americans have been killed there. As a result, many do not care to know. School boards obviously do not have a high priority in pointing out the American deaths in the Middle East, much less those of the people the soldiers killed there. Similarly, the deficiencies in education have not gotten American society very far in a basic awareness of the coronavirus and other crucial issues.

The deficiencies were there before the virus. Thus it was not unusual to go to a restaurant in pre-coronavirus days and see a family seating down for dinner (or even at home) and all of them texting throughout the dinner, without much of any conversation among them. Trump has popularized twitter with his childish rants and language throughout a given day, in one case about 100 times, and communicating in such a disjointed manner with Americans. He thus does not exemplify being a paragon of reason, and certainly not of science. He is proudly anti-scientific.

In a word, there is not much of reading that is of substance in society. Social skills have declined in society as one outcome of this. That does not bode well for comprehending the coronavirus and its ramifications, or for understanding much of anything else. In one sense, there is hope that with the protests against racism more people, especially the young, are reconsidering historical events after reading and understanding what some figures in American history really were about after all. Racist statues, mascots, songs, etc., can only be eliminated after reading history, or simply after more reading, period.

President Trump's deficiencies regarding the virus, the Middle East, race relations and many other matters are there for everyone's perusal. Yet he knows nothing of significance about education other than to repeat the mantra of DeVos (of Amway fame, his education secretary) of "school choice" articulated more by him than any comparable emphasis on public schools. Likewise, Vice President Pence had no medical expertise when he was leading the now essentially defunct task force on the coronavirus pandemic.

This is notwithstanding the non-factual, fanciful thinking of the U.S. as a peace-loving country. Even when the money was not there for these military excursions, it was provided/created through taxes with allocations by the trillions for war and therefore killing and not for life (health care, etc.). Perhaps the posturing by those in political office will now be seen for what it is.

When efforts are purported to be humanitarian there too often are political calculations involved. President Kennedy inaugurated the Peace Corps to go assist people in other countries. He did not admit the obvious, however: he did this after Fidel Castro triumphed in Cuba, and Kennedy sought to counter Castro's influence, particularly in Latin America with his Peace Corps.

Likewise, through the Marshall Plan in Europe after World War II, the U.S. sought to counter in some European countries the growing influence of the Soviet Union. Unbeknownst to the public here, the CIA moreover had in the U.S. itself hundreds of journalists to steer thinking in particular directions that the agency deemed. It was illegal.

Overall, so much was all this the case that the CIA directly toppled European governments which were allying themselves with the Soviet Union. The agency continued its involvement in assassinations in modern history, with that of Lumumba of the Congo, Diem of Vietnam, Allende of Chile, and others. A nation of laws is not the strong point after all of the U.S., whether in regard to the CIA, the racist history of the country, the pandemic today, and so forth.

The deaths and atrocities as outcomes of the illegalities are an afterthought, if that. In sum, we are a nation largely of non-readers when it pertains to substantive topics of history and other social matters, dwelling as we do on the superficialities of texting and the choppy chatter of twitter. That does not portend anything very positive for society and certainly not during a pandemic that is transforming society in myriad ways.

All this the U.S. could do because it was spared the destruction of its factories and infrastructure by World War II as happened in Europe, because of the buffers of the Atlantic and Pacific Oceans. The factories here threw out the women working when the factory owners glimpsed at the looming clouds on the horizon of insurrection/violence from the masses of unemployed soldiers returning from World War II. The soldiers stated that the humming factories had the wherewithal to hire these soldiers at good pay. Immediately the factories owners caved to their demands.

So, magnanimity has not been much in the cards in American history. The opposite has been more so the case. It is patently obvious that whatever the level of infection and deaths occur in poorer countries from the virus, no help of significance will be forthcoming from the U.S., as it has not in months of the pandemic in 2020. As a matter of fact, almost all the aid from the U.S. to other countries has been military aid, which has been outlaid to satisfy the profit-salivating weapons manufacturers here. The poor cannot eat rifles and bombs; neither can anyone else, and we need those trillions of dollars for health care, as the need has been before and as is the case now that the coronavirus infections demand it.

Khrushchev of the Soviet Union once pounded his shoe at the lectern in the United Nations proclaiming to the U.S., "We will bury you." Such a funeral turned out to be premature. The burying of so many thousands from COVID-19 is literally now the case, though, with the question remaining of how many more will die. This is not to mention the very major question of what the permeation of realistic fear and anxiety from the coronavirus will do to American society as we know it currently.

Soviet society materialized in the "ten days that shook the world" as it was termed by chronicler John Reed at the time. However, it went out with a whimper due to the unsustainable impact on their economy from the arms race. The coronavirus will do in the U.S. what no one imagined, and it is all from a virus and not war, and not in ten days that will shake the world, yet soon. Namely, the collapsing of the U.S. economy will also be with a whimper, from the aftereffects wrought by the coronavirus.

Many here jeered at the fall of the Soviet Union thirty years ago. They are not laughing anymore at what is collapsing in the U.S. Perhaps if the U.S. had not insisted on spending trillions on the arms race to supposedly defeat the Soviets in that sphere we would have been in a better position to address the coronavirus. That is not to mention the speeding up of what is collapsing around us by the racial conflict, realized now as instigated by police brutality and overall racism in the U.S. also in the spring of 2020. Clearly, one way or another, things will not be the same.

We see thus that the number of deaths from the virus are objectively higher than those from terrorism throughout the world. The coronavirus is a greater threat to the U.S. and the world than terrorism. When the number of coronavirus deaths reached about 3,000 it was stated that the virus surpassed the number killed in 9-11. When the number of virus deaths reached about 7,000 it was stated that that number was greater than the soldiers killed in Iraq and Afghanistan (of course no mention of the number of Iraqis and Afghans killed). Then when the number reached about 58,000 it was stated that the number surpassed the number of soldiers killed in Vietnam, without mentioning the countless hundreds of thousands of Vietnamese we slaughtered.

Many of those Americans, by the way, who died as mentioned above other than from the virus did so from the U.S. illegally invading other countries. International law moreover states that people in an occupied country have the right to defend themselves against the occupiers, as anyone in the U.S. would say about someone invading his or her home and occupying it. When people in those lands resist, that is not terrorism, yet the government here and the media (playing along with the U.S. government) say it is.

Terrorism, by definition, instead is when a person or persons kill people in another country to advance a political agenda. That simple and clear definition thereby includes what the U.S. has done to advance its political, not security, goals throughout the world for decades. Other definitions of terrorism obfuscate the clarity of it, such that not many people can figure out what it means.

The shifting of funding to life killing ventures for corporate benefit is gaining clarity every day for what it has been. More immediately, one of the most important outcomes of all this is not only that inequality in society has been laid bare by the triple situation blacks found themselves in regard to the pandemic, not only in they falling victim to it in greater numbers than others because of their socioeconomic circumstances due to racism, but also their greater rates of unemployment affecting them more than even before the pandemic but exacerbated by the pandemic. Their situation was given more clarity by the police killing of George Floyd, exemplifying the severe historical circumstances blacks have endured.

That leads to an ultimate consequence from all this: the baring of American history as a violent one. The racist figures in American history and similar types in Western history are now outed, one by one and from here on in. An example of this is the toppling of Onate, a Spanish "explorer" in New Mexico seen now for what he was. In the late 1500s he cut off the feet of some Native Americans to punish them, so some cut off his foot on his statue some years ago.

Similarly, Columbus long ago ceased to be admired due to his mutilations and carnage of Native Americans in North America, and on and on. Unsurprisingly, Native Americans have among the highest rates of infections from the coronavirus today, among other categories in the U.S., for the same historical and other reasons from oppressors.

Long ago Columbus and other genocidal persons should have been recognized for what they were, but they have now been laid bare and extensively so, instead of us remaining beholden to him and some others. This is a genuine education about them instead of the papering over of them by generations of history teachers, political leaders and others, many of these racists themselves.

Most do not really know much about Lincoln. His Emancipation Proclamation in 1862 was a war measure: he incorrectly hoped that slaves would revolt against their Southern slave masters and join the Union and therefore topple the Confederacy. His proclamation purposefully did not free slaves in Union states. Only supposedly freeing slaves in the Confederacy but not slaves in the Union is a non-starter on any discussion of emancipation. What he did say is that blacks were inferior to whites and he hoped they would go to Africa or elsewhere. Blacks were freed way later in 1865 only when and because the North defeated the South.

Interestingly, other countries are re-examining their colonial past, particularly European countries, and their extensive bloody assaults on native peoples. Some people in Britain are doing so. This is exemplified by Prince Harry (originally of the royal British) as it should have been centuries ago in regard to the British. Colonialism will be finally upended as it is now in the U.S. History will be seen for what it really was and is, finally, as bloodthirsty in the American and European theft of resources throughout the world. The coronavirus ultimately exposed furthermore the entrenched inequality overall in societies. Things cannot blithely continue as before.

Anxiety about the virus will not be eliminated just because Trump, for example, insists by fiat that it be so (for the furtherance of his political aspirations), or by anybody saying so. The much larger question pertains to the capsizing of the American economy by the coronavirus. Evidently that has already started with almost all commentators referring to the upending of the economy and society in general, but also in quite specific ways. The future is cloudy and uncertain in so many ways as to be almost unfathomable. Many are looking at the future with their hands over their eyes, not wanting to see what is before them. In doing that they will trip over themselves.

The corporate media does not help in these matters, well, because it is corporate. Profits matter. So much so is this the case that they seek readership or viewership for the advertisers, for the quarterly earnings for the shareholders that they serve. That which catches attention is primary, as a conveyance for the advertisers' profits. Advertisers have even admonished the media, such as newspapers, that they not place their advertisement next to gore or some such on a page, and the media have complied. The advertisers, moreover, certainly do not want the economic system questioned.

In a word their script for the coronavirus is the same as for any other catastrophe, such as a mass shooting. The media script says that the media maintain interest by producing, for example, some individual heroes and bravery to show about the ordeal. During the protests over police killings recently such media were striving to show someone cleaning up from the burnt remnants that the media emphasized were due to "outside agitators" (wrong: the great majority of whatever happened during the protesting, good or not, were from local people). Martin Luther King himself in describing, not prescribing, riots said they were the language of the unheard. Of course, the media did not quote that about him.

Thus, journalists unprofessionally report of a given situation primarily the what, when, where, and how of it, omitting the "why" they were inculcated in some journalism courses. The reason is that their editors would be loath to include the why, and thus journalists engage in self-censorship of themselves if they want to keep their job. The editor filters out what the publisher does not want. In fact, much of the "how" of the virus, such as how congregations or stadiums will maintain the six feet, if they will, is suspect in reportage, lest the institutions of society and in particular the economic come into question, as they will soon enough anyway. Corporate media do not question corporations to any significant extent. Their own profits are at stake. They are beholden to the shareholders.

The media have the technology to accomplish a lot. Still, all the fearsome technology and surveillance resources of a police state per se didn't get much traction with the determination of the protestors in so many cities, nationwide, and all in a brief period of time. This, in spite of the fact that COINTELPRO-like approaches failed as well. For those who may not be aware of such historical precedents, from the 1950s to the 1970s the Director of the FBI, J. Edgar Hoover (well-known as a racist) had a program whose acronym was derived from COunterINTELigence PROgram. For over twenty years the FBI in that program used paid agents provocateur to provoke the police, much as some unknown white individuals in protests do today, to attack protestors.

Many other methods were used to discredit and destabilize the organizing efforts of Martin Luther King and others. The media reported on much of this without admitting what the situation really was. Hoover's FBI, for example, directed that someone "neutralize" MLK. Agents certainly spared no effort to eliminate the Black Panthers when the FBI found out the Panthers had a breakfast program for black children and an after school program.

Positive things such as these by and for blacks have not been tolerated by many. This includes very importantly many whites in political office who do not seek, to this very day, to improve the health of blacks and their socioeconomic conditions and to thus decrease their coronavirus infection rates and death rates by providing health care for blacks and others. It is understandable why blacks emphasize that Black Lives Matter, because they have not mattered in the past and still do not as compared to white lives.

The media focused on the violence often from those agents of the FBI and other law enforcement agencies, much as today police infiltrators have been found to instigate violence themselves and among protestors of police brutality. The media thus discredited the social movements of the time, just as much of the media seeks today, unsuccessfully though, to discredit Black Lives Matter and other groups/movements. Some persons died as a result of COINTELPRO. That program basically failed. The FBI lost in a court case on the program. Again, the sociological axiom that things are not what they seem to be applied then during the 1960s and it applies now as well.

Again, patterns are generally much more important than what appear to be individual instances. Thus it is that the long history of violence against blacks and Chicanos has been the norm, from the slave patrols (which in practice were the earliest forms of policing against blacks) before there was the U.S.; to the Civil War over slavery; to the Black Codes following slavery; and on through to police brutality against blacks such as in Watts in the 1960s; to the police killing of a 12 year old Chicano in Dallas in the 1970s; to the police killing of a black motorcyclist in Miami in the 1980s; to the acquittal of police beating up a black (filmed) in Los Angeles in the 1990s; and to the 2000s the police brutality and riots against police in Ferguson, Oakland, Baltimore and Minneapolis, to name a few instances which follow a societal pattern for centuries.

That is not to include the ethos in police departments of antagonism against those of color, first seen in the slave patrols and to this day. Thus, all these and more are not isolated incidents and not tolerated as such anymore. This is so alongside the ahistorical framing by the media of police brutality as supposedly just isolated incidents. There are in fact in the hundreds of years just mentioned probably millions of people of color, as a pattern, who have been so treated, without any videotaping of it all as is now the case.

Likewise, today we can see the videotaped rightist infiltrators of protests, exactly as in the un-videotaped days of COINTELPRO (which many believe was not dismantled by the FBI even when ordered to do so by a court, such is the impunity of law enforcement), who still instigate violence to discredit and destabilize protest movements. Still, much of the media insists on discrediting those of color. Thus, the media is again suspect in what it reports, such as claiming that the coronavirus is spreading because of the protestors, or that the young are spreading the virus to the elderly, creating that into a generational war.

Instead the media need the history lessons on racism, genocide, etc. provided by the protestors and others. Simply put, the coronavirus and the protestors are linked and given ink by the media, instead of a focus on the macro and related aspects of the virus. With a pushback on the media about this by the protestors, the media relented and has been now reporting that the spikes in the summer of 2020 are due to the early re-opening, as Trump and others wanted for the salvation of his economy, with millions of people returning prematurely to restaurants, bars, parties, etc.

Much of the media report what happens that they consider unusual in order to grab "eyeballs" (a media term) as they did in regard to the virus, the protests, etc. Another way this is illustrated is that the media prefer the ignorance and flashiness of individual political leaders to a drab array of scientists, whether medical or social scientists. Thus, readers and viewers are not enlightened with analyses of a how a problem evolved and who the responsible parties are. The focus is on an individual or a few individuals, not the overall situation. Such atomization of a problem does not lead to its resolution as a social problem, i.e., as to why we have more crime, more health problems, less education, etc., than those in other societies.

If we did what other societies do that have the same homo sapiens born there as here, but do not anymore have the problems we do, we would be better off. Namely we then would have to have a social solution to a social problem, as they have done so in those societies when a problem emerged significantly, such as poverty. An individual solution that is proffered to a social problem is really no solution. A focus on what Trump says to the relative exclusion of scientists will not work and the COVID-19 will cause still more needless suffering and deaths as a result.

Just as the term social distance appears to be a new term, it is not. Sociology has long used it to describe types of racism. Yet the sociological term did not create an interest by the media and by society. The interest comes about in the police killing of blacks which thereafter results in images of some burning of buildings and looting. Then the media, temporarily, to save society's own skin, seeks out sociologists and other social scientists sometimes, if that. They don't often seek out social scientists, and in that sense the media is about as unscientific as the president.

The coronavirus leads to the very questioning of our economic system, given the joblessness as a consequence of mitigating the spread of the virus. Namely, the very need to buy stuff is questioned now. The very idea of the unemployed, who don't have prospects soon of a good job, buying a new car or house is ludicrous, unless of course they do so by getting into deep debt which many people so far have done. With their credit ratings now ruined, not many can even go into debt, though even in that instance there are loan sharks around the corner who will be salivating to profit from the misery of others.

Now, the macro becomes relevant, the micro less relevant. Many will practice something they did not know that there was a social science term that described it: interpersonal zones, which are the various physical distances people keep from each other depending on whether they know each other intimately or the varied and greater physical distance from others, which would depend on the circumstances. The greater distance will become the default now because of the coronavirus in almost all but the most intimate of interpersonal relationships, with society in general becoming the worse for it all. This conundrum was unexpected in recent history.

Keep in mind this is in very general terms and does address the closer relationships some may engender in others, such as in reference to race relations. Interpersonal zones do not refer either to the new social distance as defined because of the virus, nor social distance as defined in sociology for decades.

In sociology there is also what is termed blaming the victim, now in a new context because of the virus. The concept refers to when the victim of a situation, such as of poverty or of rape, etc., is blamed by society for causing the his or her own poverty or rape, in order that society can wash its hands and not deal with social problems, and thereby the status quo remains in society. Worse still is when the victim as a result comes to blame himself or herself, as well society blaming the person.

More specifically, many will blame themselves for not being exactly six feet all the time from others if they got infected and there is no conclusive science that it is exactly six feet as safe, particularly from those coughing, sneezing or talking very loud in regard to droplets scattered (as teachers and professors often have to talk louder than others and as some students do, to be heard). Some will blame themselves for not sanitizing their hands every time they handled a doorknob, or even the ubiquitous paper money.

A semblance of this is illustrated in shows such as Dr. Oz, The Doctors, and others. They imply that if the viewers do not do what they recommend, the viewers are to blame their own selves for whatever befalls them. Thus, for example, it is not pollution nor carcinogens found everywhere made by manufacturers for their own profit that are at fault for causing cancer, but the reactions of the viewers themselves in letting that happen. The admonishment is for viewers to not look at the larger picture, the macro, because if they did some things would need to be changed. The coronavirus is now forcing macro changes in society, nonetheless.

Perhaps some of these TV shows which act as a palliative for social problems should be seen for what they are. They are there as a recuperative measure, to make it possible for society to not question the macro, to focus on the micro, and all for returning to work the next day as somewhat mesmerized and malleable employees. Obviously the focus is not on the recovery of COVID-19 patients (since there would be billions spent on that), but on the recovery and recuperation of the employee from the employment anxieties in order to face the boss the next day.

Thus, as another major change that the coronavirus instituted is the push for online transactions (instead of being infected at stores by others and touching substances, etc.), which such transactions of course have soared as the virus hit the nation's economy. For workers, though, this means fewer positions needed as retail sales clerks in stores or as cashiers. To begin with, these types of positions are low pay with many female employees in particular hired for these jobs. All this now presents a problem for these low paid women, many who are now without even those types of jobs.

Still, a creation of numerous job positions for sanitizing grocery carts is not that feasible. Many grocery and other types of stores using carts are not going to be too excited were they to hire people exclusively for sanitizing the carts. That would not look good for the public, either. What they have done so far instead is sort of rotate that chore among workers in a store.

Sanitizing has been something that was done all day in a store, but the chore was done by several workers or at least not the same one. A year before the coronavirus, sanitizing carts would have appeared ridiculous to customers. Some stores recently had not even accepted returned items which may have been contaminated, though store employees may contaminate items for sale when stocking them on the shelves and at other points.

Stores have not been quite ready to hire full-time sanitizing positions in comparison to what Walmart has done in hiring full-time greeters. However, even then with Walmart there was discrimination in the hiring of older people for this rather easy job position when younger people also wanted such a job with Walmart but had not been hired for that. Of course, that is not to mention that Walmart was sued previously for not hiring enough women as supervisors, though the great majority of its workers were women. The gender factor in many issues in society is there as well.

A year before the virus there already were a very small number of customers who wore a face mask, either because they might have some illness that they did not want to transmit or because their immune systems were weak and they did not want to contract a disease from other customers, or for another reason. Other customers would look askance at such persons and perhaps move away from them. Now wearing a mask is a norm among customers, and sometimes a requirement under some circumstances when some stores and especially airlines require it. A new type of aggression has developed, that against the store employees who tell a customer he or she needs a face mask.

About the only other situations where pedestrians wore face masks were where there was a high level of pollution, such as in Tokyo and Mexico City, and there are photographs of these. Now there are designer types of masks and bandanas to place over the face for the coronavirus. Some coverings are even a fashion statement now, illustrating the evolution of some developing quandaries, or what in sociology are called emergent norms.

Equipment in a gym was not that sanitary before the virus. Now gym enthusiasts may be literally taking their lives into their own hands when they go there. Perhaps, like in the case of casino enthusiasts, they are betting high stakes that they will not get contaminated and die, and they may be right, or wrong. Again, even if they get the virus themselves asymptomatically, they may still infect their family and loved ones, a devastating scenario.

In fact there have already been cases where a person did not believe he or she would get infected (and perhaps did not wear a mask, etc.), got infected after all, and worse still it all eventuated in such member of the family infecting other members of the family. Not many can be all that confident they will not be infected. The president of Brazil in most ways was as brazen as Trump was and belittled the virus, but both got it after all. Of those who are so confident, it is a false sense of confidence in the face of the reality of the coronavirus.

Moreover, when some are fined for violating the restrictions, this may place the poor and the unemployed in a precarious situation in contrast to others. Fining is discriminatory in that some, such as certain beach goers, were fined while the "open the state" protestors, who were not practicing social distance, were not.

Also, the wealthy can pay off the fine easily. This is still another way the very coronavirus itself and the attendant restrictions go hand in hand in being more detrimental and discriminatory for some segments of society than others. Restrictions and whatnot should apply to everyone. They do not. The inequality continues unabated and more glaringly so, albeit in a new form with the virus.

Many of the above social changes are interrelated problems associated with the coronavirus. Once these changes are seen, the next steps follow logically from that. Specifically, it is not just the police that need to be defunded from their warfare weaponry, but much of the entire economy as well. This includes the unnecessary trillions squandered on the military that keep no one safe and secure, except the weapons manufacturers who are the only ones lobbying for warfare for their own profit, not for benefit of the public. Many if not most of the jobs in the military industrial complex need to be converted to where the needs are, to education, to social agencies, to health care, and so forth, a conversion of swords to plowshares, as it were, and very soon.

The coronavirus contributed to the realization by blacks that they are under deadly attack throughout society, and historically have been (including by police). Their even higher unemployment now as a result of mitigation of the virus is exemplified now in the overall precariousness of jobs for most people. All this has presaged much of the direction of the future.

It is up to everyone to articulate solutions and then to enact those solutions. No one needs to go elsewhere to live and benefit from what other societies do and experience the outcome of the social changes those societies instituted some time ago. Changes in American society have been inaugurated to some extent in the U.S. before, albeit not as pervasive and enduring and urgent as the coronavirus has now forced the hand of society.

In the 1930s major societal changes were made as well as in the 1960s, unfortunately in both cases to quell the masses. This time around the changes from the coronavirus will occur here and throughout the world. The U.S. has been (since the spring of 2020) on the threshold of major social change throughout society because of the virus.

Recommendations

There is a need for recommendations on what the direction of social change could or should be, given what the social changes are from the coronavirus. The following comprise recommendations to institute, some of which are ongoing:

Expand agencies which deal with poverty, which is likely to rise and engulf more people, stunting the development of children and causing other problems such as hunger.

State and local agencies assisting job seekers are needed more than the private ones such as Manpower Inc. Private agencies have vested interests which are not in the best interest of applicants.

Eliminate the focus on consumerism. The precariousness of employment leads to problems for those who are fooled by advertisers to buy stuff they don't need and cannot afford anymore. Mitigation of the coronavirus has made people prioritize family relationships. In a positive sense, many are now circumspect about frittering their lives away on consumerism.

Provide better education, not just more of the same type today (the online type). Online education, for example, fills a need for more education in quantity which is second class, than the first class (or at least better) classroom type which is qualitatively different. This is true for high school and college.

Concomitantly, more social science and history courses should be required at both levels of education above. One of the reasons for racial problems, for example, is the paucity of courses required in these areas, hence students do not take the courses and do not know about these and other topics, such as poverty, gender, socioeconomic class, etc. History should be revamped much more substantively than it is today, and that should have happened many decades ago. Much of history has promoted racism, sexism, and classism and it is now realized just how much of a problem it has been. Anyone who tried to change history before was reviled as revisionist, when in fact mainline textbooks were the ones which had revised and changed what had actually occurred in history. Texas even had a textbook policy of excluding material which might lead to students questioning authority, for example.

Shift billions of dollars to education and to health care from waste in the military and police departments. There is no point designating heroes subjectively in the health care field when there is nothing much done for them objectively. Other countries have recognized them objectively and those societies benefit from that.

Alongside with an increased funding in agencies and institutions of life, rather than destruction and abuse, there is a need for more staff in the former than the latter. Positions in agencies and institutions need to be paid more than they are now, which is one of the reasons many do not major in college to work in those areas, and of course there has not been much respect for such staff.

Much of this means that taxes should be increased. The public is fine with this, as citizens of other countries are, when they see the progress, the positives, etc., of their tax money going to constructive ends. They are not fine with their tax money being squandered. In fact a sticker found on cars in teachers' parking lots indicates that the Air Force should have a bake sale for a bomber they want (Congress has shoveled funding for bombers that in fact the military itself has said are not needed, and such bombers are swiftly discarded after they are built). Instead it is teachers who wind up having to take the time and energy for bake sales for knickknacks for their schools.

Lower the price of gasoline. Many saw this actually transpire during the pandemic, and they are not going to accept or be too happy about gasoline prices going up. Should they go up, then perhaps travel plans need to be curtailed to drive down the price, which is why gasoline prices went down with fewer who planned to travel during the pandemic.

Many were fine, therefore, with travel and/or vacations which were closer to home, even (local) staycations. This should be encouraged, which would also lead to less pollution and related problems. It also leads, as was observed during the spring of 2020 during the pandemic, to fewer fatalities from car wrecks.

It became clear during the pandemic that families stayed home more and mostly strengthened their relationships. They found ways to do things together, such as eating at home around the table instead of everyone scurrying about all the time.

To counteract possible tensions from cabin fever there needs to be more support for families in a positive manner, instead of only or primarily responding to family crises. Resources in this direction need to be expanded.

One of the above resources which needs to be expanded is childcare, free or affordable for all. This along with close-to-home vacations is positive for minimizing family stresses. Many Europeans enjoy paid vacations which are mandated of several weeks duration. For those who think that can't be the case here it already is, for 30 days for the military, and has been for decades.

TV shows such as Dr. Oz, Dr. Phil, and similar ones which blame the victim should be abandoned. Viewers are given the impression that they are the problem in the social problems we have. If still presented, such shows should carry a disclaimer that what is shown is only a micro situation which does not relate to the situation in society at large. That the COPS show and PD Live were ended illustrated the degraded mentality of such programs and what they in a way "taught" and normalized.

That sports at various elite colleges are being dropped for the fall is in some ways positive. They are doing so out of students' health concerns from the coronavirus. In particular, elite colleges do not need football for the financial survival of the rest of the sports programs, as other colleges do. That other colleges are dependent on football as a financial lifeblood and are instead less concerned about the very lives of their students speaks volumes about the second-class funding we have in our society for higher education. Society needs to have less violent sports and to fund higher education for all students.

Likewise is that the case with pro football, which is all about money and seethes with violence. Pro football makes a statement to rabid fans that violence as a way of life throughout the history of the U.S. and today is just fine, replete with military flyovers, etc. The rabid fans will look as they should to their own selves at games, ridiculous with masks and social distancing in stadiums, which is why they probably will not go to games, presenting an existential dilemma to the billionaire owners. Perhaps the games should be shown only on TV without the cameras panning empty stadiums, or look foolish as Trump did in Tulsa with cameras filming a mostly empty arena for his rally.

The gratuitous violence of the military, of pro football, and of the police need to be defunded, therefore. This should go without saying, but it needs to be said and recommended. The targeting of these forms of violence is ongoing now throughout society. The coronavirus sparked these discussions in a number of ways, for the better.

Journalism needs to be revamped quite extensively. Instead of focusing on the micro (the human interest tear-jerker stories), more reporting should be geared to looking at the macro, the overall problems that affect thousands or millions of readers and viewers. The reason for the micro focus is financial, which is to say that the micro catches the attention, momentarily at least, for a newspaper to be picked up and bought by a prospective reader.

If journalism is revamped to cover more so the macro, that would signify that the more meaningful would become more paramount, as should be the case. Hopefully, that would lead to more substantive reading and less of a trivial focus on texting, twitter, etc., which Trump has popularized in his twitter storms, which seems to be what he does all day long. Wouldn't you know it, he was the perfectly trivial person to popularize the trivial. He does not read, but then again neither did Bush II and neither did Reagan, all three bringing America down into to a cesspool of nonsensical thinking, often costing lives. That they were presidents says a lot about the society that elected them. In that sense we are the problem in the macro purview more than they are or were as individuals.

We should not be railroaded into a telemed and online future for some, while the better-off receive a higher quality health care and education. The telemed and online are some of the mechanisms of entrenching the inequality there is in society. It must be kept in mind that the more inequality there is in society, the more societal problems will be engendered, which is the American situation. The more equal societies have fewer societal problems.

There should be more concern with the downtrodden now that the coronavirus has shown that anybody on practically a moment's notice can be infected and perhaps even die soon thereafter. Life should be seen, and apparently is being seen now, as more precious than before, which is well and good and that should be proclaimed from the rooftops.

The greater concern for others and particularly the downtrodden should indicate now more than ever that that is what the primary mission of Christianity should be and should have been all along. Christ talked about the poor, about those in prison, the sick, the stranger who should be welcome in one's home, etc. He emphasized that, on the contrary, the wealthy would not go to heaven.

Those who are Christian therefore need to reconsider whether they need a church building and other accoutrements to practice their faith. They need to show others their faith in the way that Christ himself said: that they be known by their works. The closing of churches gave pause to many about whether going to church was all that essential. The coronavirus brought to the fore the main precept of loving thy neighbor as thyself, and that everything else was not as crucial, including those church tea socials where Christ would not have been welcome.

In a similar vein, some holidays such as Thanksgiving and Christmas should be seen in a different light than the commercial one by corporations for the latter's profit, at the cost of those subscribing to such holidays and falling into further debt. All the while, jobs are more precarious than ever and will remain so, after the widespread closings and even failures of workplaces during the pandemic. It must be kept in mind that the contingent worker is stretched to the limit and has a ruined credit rating. With the coronavirus now substantially negating the large gatherings during those and other holidays, this means that instead people should have smaller gatherings with their loved ones instead of with a mass of others that sometimes ruin what should be the closeness of most get-togethers.

Last but not least, we must soon develop a necessarily greater concern with international matters. We are all in this coronavirus pandemic together. We are interdependent with each other, as all people have been in reality throughout time.

We need to work together to resolve whatever needs to be resolved. It can be done and has been done before. The aforesaid recommendations are feasible, and in fact many are already becoming a reality as a result of the social change from the coronavirus.

Index

www.ingramcontent.com/pod-product-compliance
Lightning Source LLC
Chambersburg PA
CBHW040255290326
41929CB00051B/3381